Praise for
The No Meat Athlete Cookbook

"Clean Protein + Easy Recipes = Hot Body.
Matt Frazier rocks it all in this superstar book!"

—KATHY FRESTON, *New York Times*–bestselling author of
The Lean, *The Book of Veganish*, and *Quantum Wellness*

"Whether you're an accomplished athlete, a weekend
jogger, or someone who just wants to eat the way many of
the world's greatest athletes and healthiest people do, you've
come to the right place. If you want to look great and feel
even better, this is the book for you."

— JOHN ROBBINS, bestselling author and president of
the Food Revolution Network

"Finally, a practical, plant-based cookbook designed
for busy athletes! If you're looking to fuel your active lifestyle,
whether you're a No Meat Athlete or just interested in having
more energy and faster recovery after exercise, this cookbook hits
the spot. With an oil-free option for every plant-powered recipe,
The No Meat Athlete Cookbook is a game changer in the
health and fitness industry."

—ROBERT CHEEKE, founder and president of
veganbodybuilding.com and author of *Shred It!*

"Matt's follow-up to the highly acclaimed *No Meat Athlete*
is the perfect resource for any elite athlete or weekend
warrior looking for plant-based recipes to fuel their body.
The No Meat Athlete Cookbook provides an incredible array
of practical whole food recipes—recipes with accessible
ingredients, easy cooking techniques, and flexibility for certain
dietary restrictions, such as no-oil and gluten-free."

—BAGGIO HUSIDIC, midfielder, LA Galaxy

"From the moment I cracked it open, I was delighted
by the simplicity and spirit of *The No Meat Athlete Cookbook*.
Whether you're a hard-core athlete ready to up your game or
someone wanting to take your health and vitality to the next
level—this book covers all the bases!"

—JASON WROBEL, bestselling author of *Eaternity* and Cooking Channel host

"*The No Meat Athlete Cookbook* is filled with helpful advice for anybody interested in eating and living better, whether you're a longtime vegan or just curious about healthier food. I highly recommend this inspiring book, which will help you adopt habits to support a happy and active life."

—GENE BAUR, Farm Sanctuary president and cofounder

"*The No Meat Athlete Cookbook* is a masterpiece to behold. It is beautifully crafted, extraordinarily engaging, and absolutely brimming with sound, practical advice. The recipes are creative, fun, and wonderfully wholesome. This book provides a simple solution for everyone who is committed to healthful, compassionate choices."

—BRENDA DAVIS, RD, coauthor of *Becoming Vegan*

"Power your plate with plants and power your life! *The No Meat Athlete Cookbook* will foster your plant-based journey with creative, delicious, nutritiously abundant meals and snacks. The recipes are innovative to impress, yet practical and easy enough for everyday cooking. Whether you want to elevate your athletic performance or simply elevate your daily health and energy, this cookbook will guide and inspire you."

—DREENA BURTON, author of *Plant-Powered Families*

"*The No Meat Athlete Cookbook* is a delicious guide to making a whole-foods, plant-powered diet work for you. Based on proven medical science, it illuminates a pathway that can help you enjoy more vitality, strength, and stamina—while fighting heart disease, cancer, diabetes, and obesity. Just reading it will make you salivate. Putting it into action will help you live a long and vibrant life. Bon appétit!"

— OCEAN ROBBINS, CEO of the Food Revolution Network

"Want to turbocharge your workouts and your health? Then *The No Meat Athlete Cookbook* is your delicious guide to doing just that. It is an incredible, practical, and nutrient-packed resource."

—ROBERT OSTFELD, MD, MSC, director of the Cardiac Wellness Program, Montefiore Health System

"Meal by meal, day by day, getting your A game on track just got significantly easier with *The No Meat Athlete Cookbook!* If you want to be more active in the kitchen, in the gym, or on the trails, this cookbook is for you."

—MATTHEW RUSCIGNO, MPH, RD, plant-based nutrition expert and endurance athlete

The
NO MEAT
ATHLETE
COOKBOOK

WHOLE FOOD, PLANT-BASED RECIPES
TO FUEL YOUR WORKOUTS—
AND THE REST OF YOUR LIFE

MATT FRAZIER
and
STEPFANIE ROMINE

THE EXPERIMENT

NEW YORK

The Experiment, LLC | 220 East 23rd Street, Suite 600 | New York, NY 10010-4658
theexperimentpublishing.com

The Experiment's books are available at special discounts when purchased in bulk for premiums and sales promotions as well as for fund-raising or educational use. For details, contact us at info@theexperimentpublishing.com.

Library of Congress Cataloging-in-Publication Data

Names: Frazier, Matt, author. | Romine, Stepfanie, author.
Title: The no meat athlete cookbook : whole food, plant-based recipes to fuel
  your workouts and the rest of your life / Matt Frazier and Stepfanie
  Romine.
Description: New York, NY : Experiment, LLC, [2017] | Includes index.
Identifiers: LCCN 2016045769 (print) | LCCN 2016048593 (ebook) | ISBN
  9781615192663 (pbk.) | ISBN 9781615192670 (ebook)
Subjects: LCSH: Athletes--Nutrition. | Physical fitness--Nutritional aspects.
  | Vegan cooking. | LCGFT: Cookbooks.
Classification: LCC TX361.A8 F73 2017 (print) | LCC TX361.A8 (ebook) | DDC
  613.7/11--dc23
LC record available at https://lccn.loc.gov/2016045769

ISBN 978-1-61519-266-3
Ebook ISBN 978-1-61519-267-0

Cover design by Becky Terhune
Text design by Sarah Smith
On cover: Athlete photograph © bikeriderlondon | Shutterstock; vegetables © Ken Carlson, Waterbury Publications, Inc.;
main dish © Sarah Smith
Photograph of Matt Frazier by Bren Photography
Photograph of Stepfanie Romine by Eliza Bell Photography

All recipe photographs © Ken Carlson, Waterbury Publications, Inc.
Food styling by Sue Hoss
Prop styling by Sarah Smith

Manufactured in China

First printing May 2017
10 9 8 7 6 5

To the members and leaders of No Meat Athlete running groups
all over the world—thank you for spreading this message of sustainable,
compassionate health and fitness in such an accepting and inspiring way.

Ten percent of author royalties from this book are donated to animal sanctuaries,
including Brother Wolf Animal Rescue in Asheville, North Carolina.
Thank you for your support in helping to end the mistreatment of animals.

Contents

Stinging sweat pooled in my eyes as my vision narrowed to a dizzying kaleidoscope. I labored to catch my breath, but my chest only tightened further in response.

Eight steps up, eight remaining. Defeated by a simple staircase, I slowly awakened to a terrifying reality that I was on the precipice of the heart attack that had claimed my grandfather's life too soon.

All I could think was, *how did this happen?*

It happened because I spent the vast majority of my life hopelessly addicted to what I call *The Window Diet*—those delicious foods served exclusively through your car's driver-side window. You know what I'm talking about. Cheeseburgers and shakes. Meat lover's pizza. Buffalo wings with extra ranch. Deep-fried everything with a supersized soda to wash it all down.

It's a lifestyle that by forty had left me fifty pounds overweight and depressed—a lazy couch potato hurtling into middle age on a crash course with chronic lifestyle disease.

My staircase incident was a wake-up call.

Over the next six months, I began experimenting with food, searching for a sustainable dietary protocol that would provide me with the energy and vitality I freely enjoyed as a young person. From paleo to low carb and everything in between, I thought I had tried it all. But nothing seemed to work. Defeated, heavier, and more depressed than ever, I was ready to abandon my quest for better health. *I guess I'm just getting old.* Back to late-night reruns of *Law & Order*.

The following day, a guy named Rip Esselstyn randomly popped up on my Facebook feed. A former professional triathlete and all-American swimmer from the University of Texas, Rip had competed against me back in my swimming days at Stanford in the late 1980s. We didn't know each other well, so I can't explain what on earth compelled me to reach out.

He told me about his firefighting career and this new book he was working on called *The Engine 2 Diet*. Shortly thereafter, an advance copy arrived in my mailbox, and thus began my introduction to something called a whole food, plant-based diet. A lifestyle that promised a solution to chronic lifestyle illness with just one hitch: No more processed foods. No more animal products. Nothing with a mother. Nothing with a face. Nothing from a lab.

Extreme doesn't begin to describe what I thought of this exercise in masochism. I mean, honestly, what's left to eat? Visions of crawling across my lawn on all fours chomping on grass entered my mind.

Not for me.

My next thought turned to the grandfather I never met. Richard Spindle had been captain of the dynastic University of Michigan swimming team in the late 1920s and an American record holder who narrowly missed an Olympic team berth. In later years, he remained fit, swimming in his beloved Lake Michigan. He never smoked, nor was he ever overweight. And yet by fifty-four, he was gone.

I realized in that moment that I was fast-tracking myself to a similar fate. It was time for a leap of faith. *What happened next changed everything.*

After a mere seven to ten days of eating nothing but plants, I felt that surge of vitality I had been searching for. Out of nowhere, my energy levels skyrocketed.

Enlivened by this miraculous new lifestyle, I began working out again for the first time in over a decade. Without effort,

the extra pounds melted away. My sleep and mental acuity improved. No longer victimized by the dreaded food coma that predictably haunted me after every meal, my energy remained consistently high throughout each day. And every successive week left me fitter, stronger, and more enthusiastic about the future.

My whole life I'd been told, "Beef is what's for dinner. Milk does a body good." And yet here I was, feeling and performing better than ever without the very foods I had been told my entire life were essential for optimal health and, of course, crucial if you wanted to perform as an athlete.

Even though I had never run in a marathon, let alone competed in an Ironman, in 2008 I finished eleventh at the Ultraman World Championships—a 320-mile sufferfest widely considered to be the world's most challenging triathlon. I returned the following year to finish sixth as the fastest American.

Then, in 2010, my buddy Jason Lester and I redefined the limits of human endurance when we completed five Ironman-distance triathlons on five different Hawaiian islands in under a week—*fueled on nothing but plants.*

While I was pursuing my athletic quests in relative solitude, on the other side of the country, Matt Frazier was hard at work on his version of my story. A beautiful story he decided to openly chronicle and share when he launched *No Meat Athlete* in 2009—an authentic, personal blog that quickly blossomed into a devoted global community and the Internet's most trafficked and trusted source for all things, well, *no meat athlete*.

I can't recall the first time I stumbled onto Matt's site, but I do know that devouring every new *No Meat Athlete* post quickly became—as it has for countless others across the globe—a mandatory daily ritual in my ongoing quest for self-improvement. A virtual watercooler lifeline with Matt's knowledge, experience, and relatability serving as equal parts host and lighthouse in his readers' collective quest to live healthier, better, and more sustainably in a world spinning out of control.

Let's take stock of where things currently stand. The United States is a prosperous nation, yet we have never been more sick as a society. Seventy percent of all Americans are either obese or overweight. One out of every three Americans will die of heart disease. Fifty percent of all Americans are diabetic or prediabetic. And over half of all insured Americans are on prescription medications for ongoing chronic ailments. The heartbreaking irony? Eighty to 90 percent of these so-called chronic lifestyle illnesses are easily preventable and very often even reversible through simple dietary and lifestyle adjustments.

Freedom from our cultural addiction to meat and dairy would also mend our climate change cataclysm. Industrialized animal agriculture is decimating our environment at an unfathomable rate. Animal agriculture is the primary culprit in the destruction of rainforest habitat, contributing to mass species extinction. It's also the biggest contributor of greenhouse gas emissions, responsible for more than all of transportation combined. Moreover, raising animals on a mass scale requires an unsustainable amount of land and water, while simultaneously depleting our soil and unnecessarily polluting our oceans, rivers, lakes, and water table.

Adopting a plant-based lifestyle is the single most powerful, most positively impactful thing you can possibly do as a conscious, compassionate consumer. It's the medicine that will prevent you from becoming a health statistic. It will significantly reduce your carbon footprint. It will help preserve the earth's bounty for future generations, while sparing the lives of countless innocent animals. And, it will undoubtedly empower you to conquer even your most audacious athletic quest.

Sound like a pipe dream? Not only is it possible, it's entirely *doable*. I'm proof. Matt and Stepfanie are proof. And now it's your turn.

So set aside whatever preconceived notions you harbor. Challenge yourself and your assumptions. Let go of habits that no longer serve you. Take Matt and Stepfanie's lead and make the leap.

Packed with Chef Stepf's supernutritious, easy-to-prepare culinary delights and meal plans, in combination with Matt's sagacious step-by-step guidance and athletic experience, this magnificent book is everything you need to finally put your unhealthy food habits permanently in the rearview and adopt the lifestyle that will truly transform your life.

Over the last ten years, I have met many stewards of the wellness movement. I can honestly say that Matt is among the best there is—a rare breath of honesty, genuine integrity, and authenticity. It is with great honor that I proudly introduce *The No Meat Athlete Cookbook* to you. I genuinely hope that you will rely on this book to unleash your healthiest, strongest, and best self on the world.

May I meet you along the path.

Peace + Plants,
Rich Roll

FROM MATT FRAZIER, FOUNDER OF NO MEAT ATHLETE

We can finally say it: "Plant-based athlete" is no longer an oxymoron. Heck, these days it's not even a rarity.

That wasn't the case in 2009 when I started my blog, *No Meat Athlete*. As I wondered whether the vegetarian diet I wanted to start eating would work for marathon training and support me in my quest to qualify for Boston, a search online revealed little to calm my fears.

Stories were out there about the rare athlete who excelled *in spite of* his or her vegetarian or even vegan diet (almost nobody dared to say "because of"), but the story of plant-based diets in competitive sports lacked enough examples and any semblance of organization.

A lot has changed since then. You might even say that the plant-based fitness movement and the vegan diet as a whole have hit their stride.

Shortly after I hit "publish" on my first blog post in 2009, I caught wind of a book called *Thrive* by Brendan Brazier, a former professional Ironman triathlete who credited a vegan diet with shortening his recovery time. A few years later, *Forks Over Knives* highlighted Mac Danzig, a mixed martial arts fighter who also chose this diet to aid recovery, giving him an advantage over opponents who required more rest between workouts.

Then Scott Jurek's (*Eat & Run*) and Rich Roll's books (*Finding Ultra*) exploded onto the scene within a month of each other in 2012, both documenting the authors' incredible stories of success in ultra-endurance sports—and how that success was not *in spite of* but *because of* their plant-based diets. Jurek is an ultrarunning legend, having dominated the sport with consecutive wins at many of the world's toughest 100- and even 135-mile events, and he believes his 100 percent vegan diet played a large role in his success. And in just a few years Roll went from being a typical out-of-shape, middle-aged guy to being named one of the "25 Fittest Men in the World" by *Men's Fitness* magazine, again with the help of a plant-based diet.

At the same time, Michael Arnstein, who is known as "the Fruitarian," showed that even a raw vegan diet based almost entirely on fruit and vegetables (no nuts, seeds, grains, or oil) could work for runners. He tore up the 100-mile ultra circuit with wins at several big races, including a 12-hour, 57-minute personal best at the Desert Solstice Track Race in Phoenix—a scorching 7:45 minute-per-mile pace, then the seventh-fastest time ever by an American at the 100-mile distance.

In 2013, vegetarian triathlete Hillary Biscay dominated the women's field to win Ultraman, a grueling three-day event in Hawaii that's essentially a double Ironman triathlon. Biscay beat all other women by over three hours and finished ahead of all but two of the men!

And although the explosion really began with endurance sports (particularly ultra-endurance sports), the potential benefits of a plant-based diet to athletes have begun to reach mainstream awareness, moving beyond sports whose athletes tend to be lightweights.

In both the 2012 and 2014 Olympic games, vegetarian and vegan athletes won medals, and in the 2016 games, the only male powerlifter on the United States' team was vegan Kendrick Farris. NFL players such as defensive lineman David Carter have experimented successfully with a vegan diet. The Tour de France, the National Hockey League, and Major League Baseball have all produced stories of athletes turning to plant-based diets to get a leg up. Venus Williams even turned to a plant-based diet after being diagnosed with an autoimmune disease.

But perhaps the biggest nail in the coffin of the myth that athletes need animal protein to be strong came courtesy of Patrik Baboumian, a German strongman who broke the world record in 2013 by carrying 1,216 pounds on his back for a distance of 10 meters! And, you guessed it, he's vegan. No meat, no dairy, no eggs.

Really, this shouldn't come as such a surprise. Some of the strongest, heaviest, and most muscular animals in nature eat diets that are almost entirely plant-based. Just a few examples:

- 450-plus-pound gorillas eat a diet that is almost exclusively leaves, shoots, stems, fruit, roots, and flowers, with just 2 percent of calories coming from tiny animals such as snails and ants. (You don't see them pounding down protein shakes, either.)

- Rhinoceroses, certain species of which can weigh up to 10,000 pounds, are strict herbivores. It's nothing but plants for these big fellas.

- Elephants, some of which can be as large as 14,000 pounds, are also fueled solely by plants.

Do these animals' diets prove that a vegetarian or vegan diet is optimal for humans? Of course not. We're different animals, with different needs. The point here is simply to show that muscle mass in animals doesn't have to be the result of eating other animals' muscle.

Our species evolved through a huge variety of climates and environments, some of which provided little more than fruits and vegetables, others in which animal flesh was plentiful. As a result, we're not strictly carnivores or herbivores, but omnivores. We can survive, and even thrive, on a stunning variety of diets, and there's no better example of this than the fact that the winner of any given 100-mile ultramarathon might be vegan, fruitarian, or Paleo. In the short term, at least for fitness and moving toward an ideal weight, almost any diet based on whole foods works. (And, not surprisingly, just about any diet based on processed foods doesn't.)

So why are the athletes who choose plant-based diets doing so? Aside from ethical, environmental, or long-term health reasons (which we will cover later), recovery seems to be the big one.

It's not entirely clear how this works, and there hasn't been much in the way of formal studies comparing the performance of plant-based athletes to those who consume animal products. But what's not controversial, and what I suspect is the reason for the faster recovery reported by plant-based athletes, is most easily understood by looking at the dietary ratio of nutrients to calories.

In his number one *New York Times* bestseller, *Eat to Live*, Dr. Joel Fuhrman posits that health can be expressed as the total amount of nutrition we get (macronutrients and micronutrients such as vitamins, minerals, and phytochemicals) divided by the total number of calories we consume in order to get those nutrients. In other words, health = nutrients/calories. (It's this ratio, normalized so that the maximum is 1,000, that the popular ANDI [aggregate nutrient density index] scores— seen on the Whole Foods salad bar—are based on.) As a strong advocate for plant-based diets, Fuhrman points out that whole plants score dramatically higher on this scale than do animal products or processed food such as refined grains or oils.

So what does this have to do with athletes? Well, it's known that digestion requires a large amount of energy. And the more calories we consume, the more energy our bodies must allocate to this energy-expensive process. So if we can get all the nutrients we need to repair our muscles and cardiovascular system *in fewer total calories* with plants than we can with animal products and junk food, then we can recover more efficiently. The extra energy that we don't use for digestion can be put toward rebuilding, and the result is faster recovery. Incidentally, it's this same concept of nutrient content per calorie along with low overall caloric density that makes a plant-based diet ideal for sustainable weight loss.

The anti-inflammatory properties of plants are also crucial. While many animal products *cause* inflammation, phytonutrients and compounds in plant foods actually fight it. You've likely seen ginger, turmeric, and garlic on lists of anti-inflammatory foods, but did you know that berries, nuts, greens, and even soy have anti-inflammatory properties as well? Because tough workouts break down muscle fibers, a process that naturally creates inflammation, foods that help curb inflammation allow for faster and more complete recovery.

But if the mechanisms behind the recovery benefits experienced by athletes following a plant-based diet are still somewhat uncertain, far clearer is what this diet does for our long-term well-being and our chance of postponing or avoiding entirely the onset of the leading killers in our society—specifically, heart disease, certain cancers, respiratory diseases, stroke, and diabetes. What's more, some of the biggest killers—heart disease in particular—can actually be reversed by a whole food, plant-based diet, as Dr. Caldwell Esselstyn documented in his groundbreaking book, *Prevent and Reverse Heart Disease*.

Several ambitious and now well-known studies, including the Adventist Health Studies, the Framingham Heart Study, and the China Study (made famous by T. Colin Campbell's book of the same name), have linked plant-based diets with the prevention of heart disease and certain cancers—and in the case of the Adventist Health Studies, a plant-based diet was associated with longer life, period. Countless smaller scientific studies have shown similar reduction in risks associated with the other leading killers, and Dr. Michael Greger at nutritionfacts.org has done an excellent job of culling and presenting these findings.

Without even looking at animal rights issues or the dramatically reduced environmental impact of a plant-based diet compared with the standard Western diet, the case for a whole food, plant-based diet is a strong one. The trick, then, is in the execution—making this incredible, high-energy diet that's perfectly suited to athletes work with the rest of your life. And that's what this book and the recipes within are here for.

A Word About the Recipes

Just as my progression from omnivore to vegetarian to vegan was a steady one, much has changed about the way I eat since I wrote my first book, *No Meat Athlete*, in 2013.

That year, I trained for and completed a 100-mile ultramarathon; in the process, I discovered that when I trained harder I craved not junk food but foods closer to their natural state than what I'd eaten before. I ate fruit throughout the day, starting with my morning smoothie, cooked beans on giant salads with tahini-based dressings for lunch, and raw nuts and seeds or veggies dipped in hummus for snacks. Dinner was mostly vegetables, along with beans and grains.

I even stopped using protein powder when, out of laziness, I didn't restock the complete-protein hemp, rice, and pea blend I had been using. A week passed, then two, then a few months, until finally . . . well, nothing. I didn't notice a difference! Here I was, putting in more miles than I ever had before—my training plan for the 100-miler required me to log a 50-miler and a 50K run in the weeks leading up to the race—and I suffered no obvious consequences when I ditched the protein powder. (We'll dispel a few protein myths in Chapter 1, "Plant-Based Nutrition in a Nutshell.")

I was hooked on whole foods, and I have continued to move in that direction ever since. My family has even stopped cooking with oil at home, which is why it's optional in every recipe that calls for it in this book. The notable exception to this whole foods philosophy is immediately before, during, and after workouts, when foods that aren't quite whole—juice or even refined grains, such as the white sushi rice in Sesame-Tamari Portable Rice Balls (page 214)—are often exactly what your body needs for optimal performance and recovery.

The recipes in my first book were 100 percent vegan, and mostly whole food. But everything I know about effective and lasting habit change is based on the doctrine of "small steps." As such, those recipes are quite a bit different from what I eat on a day-to-day basis now, a reflection of the evolution of my own clean eating habits. I believe it's easier to transition to vegan if you first become vegetarian; likewise, it's easier to adopt a whole food, plant-based diet if your first foray still includes some familiar ingredients. For most people, too drastic a change is a recipe for failure, so I'm a huge proponent of the gradual transition. (For the record, it took me a year to transition to vegetarian and two more years to gradually become vegan; it has been six years since then and I am still making changes to eliminate the final traces of processed food from my diet.)

Speaking of changes and transitions, you might have noticed that I did not write this cookbook alone. For the recipes, I teamed up with my friend and fellow plant-based athlete Stepfanie Romine. She is a certified health coach and yoga teacher, as well as a trail runner, and she has written and contributed to several books on healthy living. With her background in goal-oriented health coaching and experience with creating delicious and easy plant-based recipes, "Chef Stepf" was a natural fit for this book.

We both know the challenges of balancing training with real life and believe in the importance of fueling the body for optimal performance. And that's why we've designed the recipes in this book to be adaptable, so that you can tweak them to suit your needs, depending on where you are in your whole food, plant-based progression. Think of this book as a general guide for your kitchen, with recipes to fit whatever your particular needs may be. From the foods to eat before, during, and after your workouts for optimal performance and speedy recovery to the salads, smoothies, and meals that will fuel the rest of your busy life (as well as your family's), it's all here.

This is the book, in its practicality and comprehensiveness, that I wish I'd had when I started on this diet journey eight years ago—a journey that overlapped with marathon training, graduate school, and starting a family. It's taken me that long to refine my version of the ideal plant-based diet and, just as importantly, the skills and habits that make it workable in the real world. (I confess: Parenting two young kids and running a business make the time constraints I had back then look like a piece of cake.)

Enjoy this book, but most importantly, use it! Get it dirty, dog-ear your favorite recipes, make notes in the margins, and tweak our guidelines to fit your own life. This is your playbook, so play with it! In the process, you'll be making the most valuable investment you can in the health of your family. Let's get started.

MEET CHEF STEPF (AND THE STORY BEHIND THE RECIPES)

**From Stepfanie Romine,
founder of *The Flexible Kitchen***

Back in 2010, after several years of being a vegetarian, I made the transition to a completely plant-based diet. Around the same time, I started training for my second half marathon and met my now-husband, Sam, a competitive cyclist who was commuting by bike two hours a day on top of training.

We're still running (and biking and yoga-ing) on plants. A plant-based diet has fueled me through several half marathons; it provides me with the energy I need for my six-day-a-week Ashtanga yoga practice (and my yoga teaching); and it helps me maintain my weight when I'm not training, something that's really starting to matter as I reach my midthirties. Sam bikes up to 200 miles a week during peak season.

I'm an active person, but I don't always call myself an athlete. I'm a runner, but first and foremost, I'm a yogi. I run for the solitude, the meditative benefits, and the cardiovascular boost.

Sam, on the other hand, was a collegiate rower and then started a bike team with his friends. He raced road and cyclo-cross for years, and since we moved to North Carolina he now dabbles in mountain biking, too. He has two marathons under his belt and talks of doing more. He's an athlete, for sure, and he's always pushing his body.

When I started cooking for Sam, there was a bit of a learning curve. I had cooked for crowds and was just wrapping up my first cookbook, but I had no idea how much an athlete *really* needed to eat compared with the average semiactive person. At 6 feet 3 inches and 165 pounds, he needs to consume 3,000 to 3,500 calories per day just to maintain his weight, about twice what I need. And when he rides for six hours in the mountains, he might need to *double* that amount!

The first time I fed him, I cooked a meal that I assumed would yield four servings.

He cleaned his plate in minutes, had second helpings, and finished off every last bite I had cooked. He asked: Is there dessert? My eyes widened. *He was still hungry. How was that possible?* He ended up polishing off the rest of a batch of chocolate almond butter with bananas, then ate a snack a couple of hours later.

After that night, my cooking began to change. Gone were the fussy meals with intricate components; they would be gobbled down in a few bites. I expanded my repertoire of stews, stir-fries, and bean-based meals. I learned about the specific needs of athletes versus more casual exercisers. And, very importantly, I figured out how to keep our grocery bills—and Sam's hunger—in check.

Through trial and error (and a lot of training as a health coach), I learned what fuels Sam adequately after a ride and what doesn't. I learned what sits well with me on a run and on the mat. (I've shared these tips in the pages that follow, so you can save time and money, too.)

Although I continue to cook "for fun," my repertoire is more practical than it once was, a result of years of research and experimentation with healthy, plant-based meals. I don't make complicated dishes like sushi or stuffed pastas very often; the meal will be gone so quickly that the effort feels in vain. At lunch and dinner, I always serve root veggies such as sweet potatoes or beets and usually a whole grain, too. And, because Sam can't live without it, every meal has a sauce or sauce-like component. (Chapter 8 should be dedicated to

him.) Food is well seasoned but moderately spiced to avoid GI issues on the bike or the trail the next day. It always comes in generous portions. And though I don't like sugar, I make sure we have healthy treats on hand for late-night carb cravings. There's also a great deal of inspiration from my international travels, especially from France and South Korea, both places where I lived. And since Matt and I both have lived in the Asheville area for a few years now, there's quite a bit of inspiration from the wonderful, veg-friendly restaurants here.

When we got together, word spread quickly among Sam's friends that I was a cookbook author. Most weekends, we hosted our cycling buddies for dinner and served them feasts designed to promote recovery.

Every few months for the first couple of years we lived in the mountains, those same guys would come down for a long weekend. To keep the team's costs low, I usually volunteered to cook dinner at least one night. They would give me money for groceries, and I'd whip up a huge spread. I've been the unofficial caterer at their team spring training camps, making dozens of homemade pizzas and huge pots of pasta with the other wives and girlfriends. They appreciate that not only do my meals fill their bellies, they also help them stay healthy and strong on the bike.

They kept asking for recipes so they could cook healthy meals like mine for themselves and their families. That experience feeding hungry athletes spurred the idea for Matt and me to team up and write this book.

The recipes we're sharing have been tested on real-life athletes, both pros and weekend warriors, as well as Matt's family with two young (plant-based, but still somewhat picky) children. If something gave them (or me!) "gut rot" on the bike or made a run the next day uncomfortable, it didn't go in the book.

We had food stylists and registered dietitians test our recipes, but we also had cooking newbies try them, too. Anything that got a thumbs-down was tweaked or replaced.

I've been writing about food for over a decade, and I'm thrilled to be able to work with Matt to help healthy, active people like you run on healthy, delicious plant-based meals. I hope you get as much use out of these recipes as we have, and we can't wait to hear how they help you reach your fitness goals.

A NOTE ON LANGUAGE

Now that we've each shared our stories and you've gotten to know us a bit, we're going to shift our voice to a unified "we" throughout the book (with a few exceptions we call out). We hope this helps you focus on the recipes instead of trying to figure out which one of us is "talking."

Part One

THE PREP WORK

Chapter 1

PLANT-BASED NUTRITION IN A NUTSHELL

I f you're an athlete, your diet matters as much as your training. Food fuels you. The best equipment, training plans, and coaching won't matter if your tank is empty—or you're using the wrong fuel. Whether you're a casual runner or a competitive cyclist, chances are you've experienced a bad workout. More often than not, exercise gone awry can be traced back to a lifestyle choice—lack of sleep, stress, or the wrong food (or simply not enough food).

Our goal here isn't to write a comprehensive treatise on how to achieve optimal health through plant-based nutrition.

And the good news is, you don't need that. Because (a) it's already been done—check out *Eat to Live* by Joel Fuhrman or *How Not to Die* by Michael Greger, and you'll see what we mean. And (b) to borrow a line from Bruce Lee: "The height of cultivation always runs to simplicity." In other words, 95 percent of the message you'll walk away with from any comprehensive study of plant-based eating can be summed up in just three words:

Eat. Whole. Foods.

But don't despair, we're not going to send you on your way just yet. In this chapter we'll help you feel good about such a simple approach to food and fill in most of the remaining 5 percent of the nutrition strategy by discussing protein, oil, and supplements; we'll also highlight a few of the foods that are so nourishing and protective they're worth building into your diet on a daily basis.

But first . . .

THIS IS NOT A "DIET"

At least, not in the unfortunate, mainstream, shortsighted sense of the word. Not in the "eat this way for a little while, until the next bright, shiny, well-marketed object comes along to take your focus away" sense.

In eight years of writing a popular blog and hosting a hit podcast, speaking to hundreds of experts and interacting with thousands of readers and listeners, Matt has learned one valuable lesson that transcends both diet and exercise. It's about habit change, and it's this: The positive changes you make for thirty days or three months or even a year don't matter. Not a bit, unless they continue or give way to even more positive changes.

What matters are the changes that last forever, or at least for many years—decades, even. And you've heard this before: It's not about "following a diet," it's about a creating a lifestyle, right? It's easy to pay lip service to this idea, but if you're honest, what's the lifestyle you've created around food and exercise?

Hopefully it's one you're proud of, and this book just represents the next step in your journey. But if the only "lifestyle" you've created around your health has been one of jumping back and forth between diet plans that come across your Facebook feed—avoiding certain foods at all costs one week, only to celebrate them as the new superfoods the next—then it's time for a new approach.

Forget macronutrient ratios, protein grams, and calorie counts for now. Start with the simplest of guidelines—the advice to make whole plant foods as large a portion of your diet as you can—and go from there. This simplicity, and the resultant lack of stress around food, will prove to be your greatest ally in making these changes last.

In this vein, you won't hear us say things like "Eat tomatoes; they're high in lycopene!" Because just as foods don't get better when we artificially add nutrients to them, it's a mistake to reduce whole foods to the key nutrients within them. It's *everything* in the food—and the remarkably complex interactions of countless nutrients—that our bodies thrive on, not a single constituent.

Similarly, don't get hung up on perfection, the way most "diets" tend to encourage. Small compromises help you stick with new changes and lessen the drain on your willpower as you learn to prepare new meals and navigate social situations centered around food.

When it comes to diet changes, there's an unfortunate tendency toward perfectionism—every meal must be perfect, with no slip-ups and no "cheating." And that means when the inevitable deviation happens (giving in to a craving or even just neglecting to plan ahead), we feel as if we've failed, and often go back to our old ways.

Instead, be OK with small compromises. If your motivations for eating a plant-based diet are rooted mostly in ethics, then you probably won't want to make occasional allowances and eat animal products. But this doesn't mean you can never, ever eat "vegan junk food"—every now and then, it's a fun treat! And if a little bit of flexibility is what keeps you on track the other 95 percent of the time, then it's a good thing. Even Dr. Fuhrman, viewed by many as fairly strict among the "vegan docs," writes that in the research he's done, he can't tell if there's a difference from a health perspective between a perfect diet and one with up to 10 percent of its calories from junk food (and for Fuhrman, junk food includes animal products, refined carbohydrates, and oil).

The recent controversy over the merits of fruit and vegetable smoothies demonstrates the "small compromises" point well. A vocal contingent in the plant-based community has pointed out (accurately) that it would be more natural to eat whole and unblended fruits, vegetables, nuts, and seeds than to blend them into a drinkable smoothie. We'd eat fewer calories this way, since it would take more effort and more time to chew the food and the increased volume would take up somewhat more room in our stomachs than a liquid smoothie would.

If the goal is extreme weight loss, we understand their argument. For most athletes, though, that's not the goal, and in fact, many plant-based athletes focus more on making sure they get *enough* calories than on limiting them. But the bigger problem is that for nearly everyone—and *especially* for those at the very beginning of their healthy-eating journey—the choice of what to eat for breakfast on a busy morning isn't one between a smoothie and a bowl full of raw fruits, vegetables, nuts, and seeds! Most people simply aren't going to eat the latter for breakfast, at least not until they've become quite accustomed to eating this way over several years. The more typical decision for someone new to healthy food is between a smoothie and something that comes out of a drive-through window . . . or in a better scenario, between a smoothie and bagel. The bagel isn't so bad if it's whole grain and unprocessed—but compared with the micronutrient powerhouses that are raw fruits, vegetables, nuts, and seeds? We'll take the smoothie any day, even if it's not quite as good a choice as the unblended ingredients would be if we could get ourselves to eat that way every day. Most of us can't, or won't, and by recognizing our own limitations, we can remove a tremendous amount of the stress connected to diet.

THE WHOLE FOOD, PLANT-BASED PHILOSOPHY

A simple formula for health, as much as there is one, comes from Dr. Fuhrman: Health equals nutrients divided by calories ($H = N/C$). In other words, the more micronutrients you can get in the fewest number of calories, while still eating whole foods, the healthier you'll be. (Of course, the assumption here is that the total number of calories is within a reasonable range—enough to thrive but not more than you need to support your metabolism and activity level.)

Notice that there's no explicit exclusion of animal products there, by the way. But because "whole" animal products are calorically dense and relatively low in micronutrients, they typically score pitifully low on the H = N/C scale compared to plants.

Although "health" in this context typically means remaining at or moving toward your ideal weight in the short term, and protection from (or even reversal of) disease and inflammation in the long term, it might just explain why so many top-level athletes are turning to plant-based diets to speed recovery from workouts. From a health perspective, lots of micronutrients in relatively few calories means your body gets lots of the raw materials it needs to repair and protect itself, without having to do excessive work (and creating excessive waste) in the way of metabolizing calories. The same reasoning applies from an athletic perspective, where the focus is on repairing your body from tough workouts: When you feed your body lots of nutrients without a lot of empty calories, very little work (or time) is required to use them. The result is your ability to complete more workouts per week than the competition— or for those of us who don't necessarily want to increase our workout frequency, it simply means showing up to your next one fully recovered and ready to do it all again.

Of course, just because a food doesn't contain any animal products doesn't mean it's healthy. There's plenty of vegan junk food in the world these days, and while that's a fun change of pace compared with even just a few years ago, it's not going to help your body stay healthy or recover quickly from workouts.

In addition to being plant-based, food should also be whole. That means refined flours and added sugars (white flour, white rice, maple syrup, agave nectar, cane sugar, etc.) are out—at least from a 100 percent whole food diet. The same goes for oils, even supposedly healthy choices such as olive, coconut, or grapeseed oil (more on this in a bit). Again, this isn't to say you can never or should never have them if that small allowance every now and then will help you to establish habits that last for years, not months. Remember the 10 percent rule, and keep the non–whole food calories in your diet below that threshold. (You'll see that we use a few not-quite-whole foods sparingly in our recipes, especially in those meant to be athletic fuel, where processed carbohydrates are more readily available for the body to use than whole food forms.)

This is also why smoothies are better than juice. When you juice fruits and vegetables, you remove more than just the fiber. You also remove the nutrients that bind to fiber, so you lose micronutrition (and the integrity of the whole food) while increasing caloric density. Blend the whole fruit into a smoothie, though, and you've got everything that's in the whole fruit, in a convenient, on-the-go form that lets you add even more whole food nutrition to your diet.

BUT . . . WHAT ABOUT PROTEIN?

If you're new to this diet like most people, we know what you're thinking: Where am I, an athlete, going to get my protein? In a world hell-bent on getting its protein (and spurred on by advertisements and big-agriculture lobbyists), we know this next bit is going to be hard to believe.

If you eat whole foods, you don't need to worry about getting enough protein. Even when those foods are plants.

Take a look at the elite athletes who excel on a plant-based diet. Remember Michael Arnstein, who ran 100 miles in under 13 hours (a sub-8-minute-mile pace)? In his diet of raw fruits and vegetables, only about 10 percent of the calories are protein. Other vegan athletes such as Brendan Brazier and Scott Jurek have said that they get roughly 15 percent of their calories from protein, and even Chris Carmichael (Lance Armstrong's nutrition coach for many years) recommends in his book *Food for Fitness* that most endurance athletes—omnivores and vegans alike—get just 12 to 15 percent of their calories from protein for optimal performance.

So what type of diet gets you in this range? You guessed it: a whole food, plant-based one. Over 25 percent of the calories in most beans comes from protein, with chickpeas, lentils, and soybeans being more than 30 percent protein. Almonds are 15 percent protein; whole wheat is 14 percent. Most fruits contain less protein than these foods, but take a look at some common vegetables: 34 percent of broccoli's calories are protein; kale is 35 percent protein. And Popeye was onto something with spinach: *Over half* of its calories are from protein.

So you can see that it's not just tofu, beans, and nuts that pack the protein in a plant-based diet. Indeed, just about everything else in whole food, plant-based diets—grains, veggies, everything except most fruit—has a protein content at or above 12 to 15 percent of the total calories. Put it all together, and you get a diet that provides you with plenty of protein—even as an athlete.

The trick here, of course, is to eliminate most processed foods from your diet. These foods have much of their protein (not to mention fiber and valuable micronutrients) removed. Sugar and oil won't give you any protein, and the more of these foods you include in your diet, the more you bring down the average amount of protein. So yes, if you were to eat a vegan diet loaded with junk food, maybe it's true that you wouldn't get enough protein to meet your athletic goals. But if you base your diet on whole foods, you'll likely consume an adequate amount of protein with little effort.

OK, so we can clearly get enough protein from a plant-based diet—but what about the quality of that protein? Aren't animal proteins better because they're "more complete" than plant proteins?

It used to be thought that because some plant foods contain relatively low amounts of certain essential amino acids (that is, amino acids that our bodies can't produce and thus we need to get from food), plant foods with complementary amino acid profiles needed to be combined within a single meal—rice and beans, for example. As it turns out, the need to combine proteins is a myth that was debunked back in the 1990s; yet for some reason it persists to this day. Instead of using only the amino acids from the most recent meal, our bodies pool amino acids and recycle proteins already in the body so that, according to Dr. Greger, it's "practically impossible to even design a diet of whole plant foods that's sufficient in calories but deficient in protein."

And as if that weren't enough, it turns out that by eating all that animal protein you've been told you need to consume, you might be actually courting disease and inflammation. Certain animal proteins—complete proteins in particular—have been shown to increase our bodies' levels of insulin-like growth factor 1 (IGF-1), a hormone linked to colorectal, prostate, and breast cancers. Growth in the gym is one thing—and yes, animal proteins might help you achieve it—but if it comes at the cost of an increased risk of cancer? No thanks.

As you might imagine, all of this information certainly debunks the idea that you need a protein powder (most of which aren't whole foods anyway) in your diet. That said, a powder can be very helpful psychologically, when you're new to this diet and worried about protein, especially when everyone around you is saying you won't get enough. It could also be useful later as a convenience food or to help fit your plant-based diet into other nutritional philosophies that may rely on higher protein intake.

CALORIE DENSITY: THE KEY TO HEALTHY WEIGHT (AND THE ANSWER TO "WHY NO OIL?")

A striking difference between this book and Matt's first one, *No Meat Athlete*, is that every recipe in this one is oil-free or includes an easy oil-free option. So what's the deal with oil?

Even a cursory glance at the books and documentaries in the plant-based nutrition world turns up doctor after doctor (Neil Barnard, T. Colin Campbell, Caldwell Esselstyn, John McDougall, Fuhrman, and Greger, to name a few) discussing the benefits of a "whole food, plant-based diet." Oil is such a part of our culture's cooking that it's easy to assume that oil (especially the much-lauded extra virgin olive oil) is healthy and whole. But a closer look reveals that when vegan doctors talk about whole foods, oil is not one of them.

Coconut, sure. Coconut oil, no.

Avocado, wonderful. Avocado oil, not so good.

Olives, you bet. Olive oil, not the health food it's cracked up to be.

Oil is the fatty part of what was a whole food. When the oil is pressed out, it brings with it many of the calories but leaves behind most of the valuable micronutrients in the plant it was removed from. Lots of calories, not many nutrients: In other words, oil doesn't score high on the H = N/C scale.

But there's an even bigger reason to think twice about drizzling olive oil on your salad, or starting your onion and garlic sauté by taking your oil bottle for few laps around the pan. And that reason is calorie density, which may just be the most important secret to a healthy weight and athletic performance.

We're used to thinking about food in terms of calories per serving. But just for comparison's sake, let's take a look at the number of calories *per pound* of some common foods.

Of course, nobody in their right mind consumes a pound of oil (or a pound of almost anything) in one sitting, but this demonstrates how poorly oil fits in with foods that are truly whole—it's over 40 percent more calorically dense than nuts and the seeds, and over 400 percent more dense than the next whole food (avocado) up the list!

For people aiming to lose weight, this is critical. The more calorically dense a food is, the less room it takes up in your stomach, so the more calories you'll need to eat before you feel full. If you're eating foods from the top half of the list, a stomach full of food might comprise 500 calories, maybe 700 if you go really big. But you can see how including foods from the bottom of the list, particularly oil, would make it easy to fit 1,000 or more calories into your stomach with the same level of satiety.

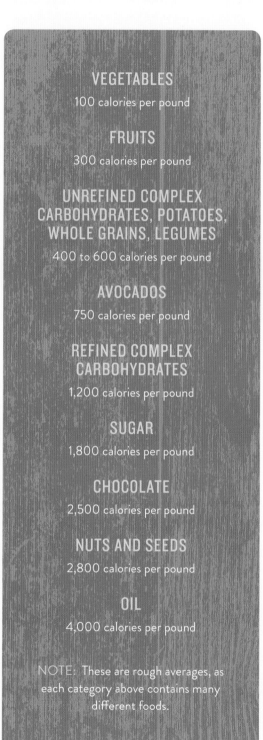

VEGETABLES
100 calories per pound

FRUITS
300 calories per pound

UNREFINED COMPLEX CARBOHYDRATES, POTATOES, WHOLE GRAINS, LEGUMES
400 to 600 calories per pound

AVOCADOS
750 calories per pound

REFINED COMPLEX CARBOHYDRATES
1,200 calories per pound

SUGAR
1,800 calories per pound

CHOCOLATE
2,500 calories per pound

NUTS AND SEEDS
2,800 calories per pound

OIL
4,000 calories per pound

NOTE: These are rough averages, as each category above contains many different foods.

So to lose weight, just stick to foods that are near the top of the list, in the top three or four slots. You can eat those until you're completely full, whenever you're hungry, and you'll likely find that your body moves quickly toward its ideal weight. (This also applies to those of us trying to maintain our weight as we age.)

If your goal is to gain weight, the same principles apply, but you'd want to consume lots of foods (still whole, in order to do it healthfully) that are fairly dense in calories—you still don't want to miss out on the micronutrients that fruits and veggies provide, but you'll find it easy to get lots of calories if you focus on calorie-dense foods such as sweet potatoes, beans, avocados, nuts, and seeds.

To this point, there are some really healthy foods such as nuts and seeds that are calorically dense. Especially if they're raw, nuts and seeds pack lots of micronutrients into their calories, and they are strongly linked to longevity. The only reasons to consider avoiding nuts, aside from an allergy or intolerance, would be if you're trying to lose weight, reverse heart disease, or are at high risk for developing heart disease, and even then it's not entirely clear that the risks of eating nuts outweigh the benefits.

Like other diet changes (assuming you don't have a dire health situation), eliminating oil is one to take on gradually. A long drizzle of oil several times around the pan to begin cooking a meal can become a ta-blespoon. Before long, you can reduce that to a teaspoon or two. Even if you have no desire to completely ditch oil, try lessening it in a gradual fashion like this to see just how little you miss it.

A final note on oil-free cooking: Since oil consumption isn't typically an ethical issue like the consumption of animal products is, you may not need or want to remove every drop of added oil from your diet. And that's OK. Matt's family doesn't often use it at home anymore (and they cook 90 to 95 percent of their food at home), so they get most of the benefits of eating this way without having to feel like they can never eat a really special meal made with oil. Stepf isn't oil-free and has no plans to be, though she does try to limit it in her recipes.

As we said earlier, every recipe in this book is either oil-free or includes an easy oil-free option, and we hope that if you've been curious about cooking without oil, the recipes here will make it easy for you to give it a try without sacrificing much in the way of flavor.

In rare cases, we use store-bought ingredients that may contain oil. You have the choice to omit certain parts of a recipe to keep it 100 percent oil-free, such as the crust in the No-Bake Mocha Cheesecake (page 258), or swap in an oil-free version of the ingredient, such as using chipotle chile powder in the Chipotle–Pumpkin Seed Salsa (page 243).

If you follow a strict oil-free diet, be sure to read the labels of any store-bought

FOODS
WORTH EATING
Every Single Day

This list started as an article on the *No Meat Athlete* blog, and it quickly became a reader favorite. It has changed over time, but the foods here are the ones we actually do try to eat every single day for their health benefits. More importantly, we explain *how* we make sure to eat each one.

You'll see that incorporating these foods daily (or any food you want to eat daily) is like creating any other habit. They must be built in to your routine, so that you don't need to make a special effort to eat them; it happens automatically. (Note that many can easily go into a smoothie, and many can easily go into a salad—a big reason to build your diet around these two meals!)

1

FRUITS, ESPECIALLY BERRIES

HOW TO GET THEM DAILY:
A few handfuls in a smoothie, first thing in the morning. We almost always use frozen berries—which aren't much different from fresh in terms of nutrition—but when they're in season and we can get them at the farmers market or from the farm, we'll use fresh.

. . . . . .

Strawberry Shortcake Rice Bites (page 216)

. . . . . .

Blueberry-Walnut Vinaigrette (page 155)

2

LEAFY GREEN AND CRUCIFEROUS VEGETABLES

HOW TO GET THEM DAILY:
Salads, smoothies, and sautéed as a side

. . . . . .

Colcannon (page 164)

. . . . . .

Lemony Steamed Kale with Olives (page 161)

. . . . . .

Almost Instant Ramen (page 116)

3

NUTS AND SEEDS

HOW TO GET THEM DAILY:
Use 1 to 2 tablespoons per smoothie or salad.
Our favorites: flaxseeds (be sure to grind them), chia seeds, pumpkin seeds, walnuts

. . . . . .

Chipotle–Pumpkin Seed Salsa (page 243)

. . . . . .

Banana Cream Chia Pudding Parfaits (page 249)

. . . . . .

Emergency Vegan Shakin' Bits (page 247)

. . . . . .

Crazy Mixed-Up Nut Butter (page 57)

4

TURMERIC—AND OTHER HERBS AND SPICES

HOW TO GET THEM DAILY:
In just about everything you eat! Add flavor to salad dressings, cooked grains, and even smoothies (cardamom, basil, or cinnamon). For turmeric specifically, try:

......

Sesame-Turmeric Oven Fries (page 173)

......

And check out Chapter 8 for all our "Flavor Boosts" with herbs and spices.

5

BEANS

HOW TO GET THEM DAILY:
In a wrap with veggies for breakfast, sweetened for a snack, in a dip such as hummus, and as the base for your dinner

......

Slow-Cooker Refried Beans (page 174)

......

Bulked-Up Smoothie (page 201)

6

ONIONS AND GARLIC

HOW TO GET THEM DAILY:
As the foundation of flavor for every dish you sauté!

......

Quick Pickled Onions (page 240)

......

Roasted Garlic Dressing (page 148)

7

MUSHROOMS

HOW TO GET THEM DAILY:
By sipping on homemade mushroom broth, sautéing them for your morning tofu wrap, or in stir-fries. (Mushrooms should be eaten cooked, not raw, as they contain toxins that are deactivated when cooked.)

......

Better than Bone Broth (page 210)

......

Shiitake Bakin' (page 62)

8

GREEN TEA

HOW TO GET IT DAILY:
During an afternoon break from work—either brewed hot or iced from the fridge (the leaves are good for three infusions)

......

Frozen Matcha Latte (page 199) with Sweet Red Beans (page 253)

......

Slow-Cooker Coconut-Matcha Brown Rice (page 47)

OTHER FOODS TO EAT SEVERAL TIMES A WEEK

Though the above foods are the ones worth designing your daily food habits around, there are many others that fill out a varied plant-based diet. You'll see that these foods also show up in a lot of our recipes.

1 Avocado (often on toast or in place of dressing on a salad)

2 Coconut products (coconut butter or manna, coconut milk)

3 Ginger (sometimes as tea and in smoothies or stir-fries)

4 Tomatoes (raw in salads or cooked in stews and main dishes)

5 Lemon juice (to brighten up a dish)

6 Dates (usually as fuel during a run, or in treats)

7 Dark chocolate (as a treat)

ingredients, such as salsa, marinara sauce, hot sauce, and chocolate chips.

And with pancakes and waffles, you have two options: Use a well-seasoned skillet or waffle iron that does not require oil, or opt for a small amount of oil or cooking spray to keep your pancakes and waffles from sticking.

A WORD ABOUT SUPPLEMENTS

We've explained why protein supplements are unnecessary for almost everyone. But that's certainly not to say you should write off supplements entirely. Before we go into detail, however, it's important to understand that your needs might be different from ours, so don't assume that because we take (or don't take) something, that you'll want or need to do the same. We recommend talking to a doctor, nutritionist, or registered dietitian about supplementation. Our goal for this section is to give you a place from which to start asking questions.

First: Vitamin B12 is as close as you'll find to a universally recommended supplement for those eating 100 percent plant-based diets, so that's one we highly suggest. Vitamin B12 deficiency is quite common, even among omnivores, and B12 is very hard to come by in a plant-based diet, with the exception of foods that are fortified with it. Some vegans argue that because B12 comes from a bacteria found in the soil, we can get it without supplementation just by eating "dirty" produce; this same argument is used in defense of the plant-based diet when the lack of B12 is cited as evidence that it's not natural to eat only plants. Perhaps produce, before it was washed as thoroughly as it is today and when soils were healthier, provided all the B12 we needed. But we're not convinced, and we like to wash our vegetables. So we take B12 in our multivitamin and recommend that you do, too.

This raises another question: If you can find standalone B12 supplements, apart from an entire multivitamin, why take the multi?

We're all for whole foods, and with a varied diet you can probably get most of what you need. But as a safeguard, we like to take a multivitamin. Aside from the fact that the poor quality of modern soil and other modern agricultural practices make the nutrient content of fruits and vegetables lower than those we evolved to eat, there are several nutrients that are commonly deficient in 100 percent plant-based diets. According to Dr. Fuhrman in *Super Immunity*, these are:

- Vitamin B12
- Zinc
- Iodine
- Vitamin D
- Vitamin K2
- Omega-3 fatty acids

We should point out that mega-doses of vitamins, minerals, and other nutrients can be dangerous. Even vitamins that were long thought to be safe in high doses have turned out not to be; an example is vitamin A, which in large doses has been linked to cancer. To limit the chance that your multivitamin does more harm than good, look for one derived from quality sources and that contains relatively small doses.

Of the nutrients in the list above, all but omega-3s can commonly be found in multivitamins. But surely we can get omega-3s from walnuts and flaxseeds, right?

Not so fast. The catch is that omega-3s comprise three types of fatty acid (alpha-linolenic acid [ALA], docosahexaenoic acid [DHA], and eicosapentaenoic acid [EPA]) and plant foods typically provide just one of them.

People (not just vegans) are commonly deficient in all three types, but ALA is quite easy to get in walnuts, seeds (hemp, flax, chia), and leafy greens. This, plus the general link between nuts and longevity, is the reason these foods are a great addition to smoothies.

But DHA and EPA are harder to find in plant foods. And it turns out that although some people's bodies are able to convert ALA into DHA and EPA in sufficient amounts, others cannot. For this reason, you should add a DHA/EPA supplement to your smoothie or water each morning. A blood test can determine whether your body is capable of converting enough ALA into DHA and EPA, but if you're not going to get tested, it's probably worth taking a supplement to be safe.

Chapter 2

YOUR PLANT-BASED KITCHEN

Whether you're running a marathon or cooking dinner, all the knowledge in the world won't help you if you don't put it into practice. But all too often, exotic ingredients and complicated techniques create a roadblock in the kitchen, especially for busy athletes. We both like to cook for fun, often with our spouses. But most nights, after a day of work and at least one workout, we are hungry and tired (and, admittedly, sometimes hangry) at dinnertime. We don't want to spend an hour in the kitchen or deal with a sink full of dirty dishes before bed. And when faced with a choice between perfectly pan-seared tofu that requires our undivided attention or baked tofu that's nearly as crisp and requires far less supervision, we'll choose the hands-free option. (We think you probably would, too.)

Throughout the book, we chose ingredients and methods that strike a balance between quick and flavorful. We streamlined our choice of spices, nixed steps that required dirtying an extra pan, and chose cooking methods that require less hands-on work. The result: really good food that works in real life. We developed these recipes out of necessity and a desire to feed ourselves nourishing, satisfying food while balancing training with the rest of our busy lives. After months and years of having them in regular rotation, we decided to write this book. But before any dish made the cut, it was tested on busy nights by people like you—those who are trying to get food on the table in a reasonable amount of time. If a recipe took too long or seemed too complicated, we eliminated it.

Before we start cooking, let's look at how you can stock your kitchen to make meal planning and prep a little easier. We'll give you a peek inside our No Meat Athlete kitchens and share our must-have supplies, time-saving cooking techniques, and tips.

STOCKING THE NO MEAT ATHLETE KITCHEN

As we drafted a kitchen "must-haves" list, we couldn't think of a single item in our kitchen that is used for just one purpose, aside from our coffee- and tea-making supplies. Sure, you could buy an avocado scoop if you really want one, but you won't find it on our list of essentials. Here are the No Meat Athlete kitchen must-haves, many of which you may already have at home:

GOOD KNIVES: Don't worry about buying a full set; all you really need are an 8-inch (20 cm) chef's knife and a paring knife. They don't need to be fancy or expensive, just make sure they are sharp and continue to stay that way. Your chef's knife will handle all your slicing and chopping needs, so you'll use it daily. It should feel comfortable in your hand, with a sturdy handle and a thick bolster (the metal that extends from the blade's edge to the handle) that will serve as a finger guard. Your paring knife should be 3 or 4 inches (7.5 to 10 cm)

in length, with a blade that extends through the handle. (Skip the ceramic versions, which can chip and break.) You'll use this for detail work, such as trimming or peeling fruits and vegetables.

Y-PEELER: A Y-peeler does the same job as the traditional veggie peeler, but it's shaped differently. Instead of the blade being an extension of the handle, it's perpendicular to it, attached by a "Y" shape. The Y-shape and sturdy construction make it much easier to use! Believe us: It is a worthwhile investment, allowing you to peel vegetables in half the time—you can zip up and down rather than having to go back to the end and start over. Peel the usual suspects like carrots, beets, and parsnips, as well as butternut squash and mangos. (Keep the fingers of the hand that's holding the food out of the path of the blade—it's sharp!)

TIP: *Use your peeler to make vegetable noodles without a spiralizer. The peeler will make ribbon-shaped pasta that resembles pappardelle.*

LARGE CUTTING BOARD: Sure, you could use a bunch of little bowls to hold each ingredient, but we much prefer using a cutting board instead. Choose one that's large enough for you to chop in the middle and front, then move each ingredient to the back while you finish your prep. Transfer the ingredients straight from the cutting board to your pan.

TIP: *You can use your knife to collect your chopped ingredients, but use the top of the knife—not the blade side. Scraping the blade along the cutting board will cause it to dull. Even better: Invest in a bowl scraper with a flat edge. You can use it to clean out your bowls or food processor and clear your cutting board.*

BLENDER: We highly recommend purchasing a high-speed blender, such as a Blendtec or Vitamix. We've burned through enough cheap blenders and suffered through enough chunky smoothies and gritty cashew cream to make the investment in one of these high-end models worthwhile. Look for sales at places such as Costco or opt for a refurbished model that comes with a warranty. It will pay for itself within a year—ours both did. We use them daily for everything from smoothies to cashew cream.

TIP: *If the blender you choose offers additional parts, opt for the additional dry blade container (you can save big by grinding your own whole grains, legumes, and nuts) and the single-serve container (it makes smoothies a breeze).*

FOOD PROCESSOR: This is a busy cook's BFF, hands down. A heavy-duty model with a weighted bottom and stronger motor—such as a Cuisinart—can handle everything from slicing beets and shredding sweet potatoes to combining ingredients for veggie burgers. While a high-speed blender is better for making hummus, nut butter, and pesto, the food processor can't be beat when it comes to prepping vegetables. When we make soups, stews, and slaws, we use the slicing and shredding blades for everything from onions to cabbage. Though we could do these tasks by hand, we love the quick, even results a food processor provides. If you aren't ready to invest in a heavy-duty model, even an entry-level food processor will do.

TIP: *If a recipe has a lengthy ingredient list, such as vegetable soup, use the food processor to prep each item in the order it will be used, then transfer it to the pot as needed. This saves so much time!*

GLASS STORAGE CONTAINERS: If you're going to pay attention to what you put in your body, it's important to know that how you store and reheat your food matters. Since plastic—even items touted as "BPA-free"—can leach harmful, hormone-mimicking chemicals into your food, glass is a safer choice. Glass containers cost more up front, but they last for years, clean up easily, and can go from fridge to microwave; many are even oven- and dishwasher-safe. Pyrex has an affordable ten-piece set, and for most people, two sets should suffice.

TIP: *Hand-wash the lids to prolong their lives and keep them from warping or cracking in the dishwasher.*

CANNING JARS: These jars might be the hip and trendy way to serve drinks and food these days, but we like them because they are also practical and affordable. The half-pint (240 ml) jars are useful for storing spices and sauces, while the quart-size (950 ml) ones are ideal for taking salads, juices, and smoothies on the go. You can buy them by the dozen at most large supermarkets year-round.

TIP: *You can even take canning jars to the store to avoid using plastic bags for bulk items. Weigh them first and write the weight on the bottom of the jar in permanent marker.*

BAKING SHEETS: One of our favorite time-saving tricks is to use the oven whenever possible, especially for cooking vegetables. Baking and roasting don't require as much supervision as sautéing or simmering do. For this, baking sheets are incredibly useful. You'll only need two, since that's how many can fit in most ovens at any one time. Buy baking sheets that are rimmed, which will help prevent food from sliding or rolling off.

SILICONE LINERS OR MATS: These mats are used to line baking sheets and prevent food from sticking; they are especially helpful for oil-free baking and roasting. After experimenting with quite a few types of silicone pan liners over the years, we have determined that the original Silpat brand from France is by far the best. These mats are also the most expensive, but they hold up well and wash easily. You'll only need two, and they'll last for thousands of uses.

TIP: *To make cleanup from baking or roasting even easier, use parchment rather than a reusable liner. We prefer the un-*

bleached variety. To reduce waste, save parchment for busy nights when you need to streamline your cleanup or for items such as veggie burgers, where you will reuse the parchment for storing. (Cut it and place a piece between each burger.)

MEASURING CUPS AND SPOONS: To ensure you get the desired results from any recipe, you'll need to use measuring cups and spoons. Choose durable stainless steel varieties with clearly marked measurements that won't rub or wash off. You'll also want a measuring cup especially designed for liquids.

BAKING DISHES IN VARIOUS SIZES: We rely heavily on the oven for one-dish dinners. Choose small 1.5-quart (1.5 L) casserole dishes with a lid for vegetables and whole grains; the 3-quart (3 L) versions are great for casseroles and full meals. A 9 by 13-inch (23 by 33 cm) baking dish is also useful for lasagna and layered dishes. We prefer ceramic or enameled cast iron to glass, but the choice is yours.

TIP: *No lid? Instead of using aluminum foil to cover a 9 by 13-inch (23 by 33 cm) baking dish, invert a baking sheet and use it to cover the top. It fits well and is easier to remove if you need to check the progress of a dish.*

SKILLETS: Ideally, you should have a large cast-iron skillet and a nonstick ceramic one, but if your cast-iron skillet is well seasoned and properly maintained, that's all you need. From sautéing vegetables to making pancakes, a nonstick pan is incredibly useful, especially if you eat and cook oil-free.

DUTCH OVEN OR HEAVY-BOTTOMED POT WITH AN OVENPROOF LID: It can double as a stockpot and is great for soups, stews, and sauces. We love the enameled cast-iron ones, but any heavy pot with a lid will do. Choose one that's at least 5 quarts (5 L).

MESH STRAINER: A sturdy metal mesh strainer is far more versatile than a plastic one. All the concerns about plastic leaching chemicals into food make us feel a little nervous to drain hot liquid through plastic. Use it to drain and rinse beans, wash produce, strain stocks, drain pasta, and thaw vegetables.

SALAD SPINNER: A good salad spinner means the difference between a perfectly dressed salad and a soggy one. It can also be used to dry fresh herbs, which will stick to your knife and spoil faster if they're water-logged. If you are eating greens daily, this almost single-purpose tool is absolutely worth it.

COOKING TECHNIQUES TO MAKE YOUR LIFE EASIER

What stands between a lot of people and a healthy, home-cooked meal is actually knowing how to cook. While we can't help you become a Michelin chef, we can help you get comfortable in the kitchen. You'll love the feeling of self-sufficiency that comes with preparing your own meals.

Here's a quick primer on some of the most common techniques we'll use. Don't worry if you don't know *braise* from *broil* (or don't care to learn); we offer step-by-step directions in every recipe.

BRAISE: Slow-cooking food—such as vegetables, beans, tofu, or tempeh—in a small amount of liquid (usually water or broth). You can add aromatics such as carrots, onions, or garlic, as well as a bit of acid such as wine, vinegar, or citrus juice, to keep the vegetables from turning to mush and add extra flavor. Braising can be done on the stovetop or in the oven, and it helps dishes develop more flavor without oil. This technique is best used for beans and hard vegetables, though delicate vegetables and fresh herbs can be added at the end.

BROIL: Cooking food under direct heat to brown it. Broiling essentially produces the same results as grilling, though the heat source is on top instead of below. This technique works well for foods that cook quickly, such as tofu, bell peppers, and eggplant.

ROAST (AND BAKE): Roasting and baking are essentially the same technique; the only real difference is oven temperature. Baking is gentler with lower oven temperatures—350 to 400°F (180 to 200°C)—and results in little to no browning. When baking, dishes can be covered or uncovered.

Roasting typically requires a temperature of at least 400°F (200°C); the increased heat concentrates flavor and promotes browning. With roasting, dishes are not covered.

SAUTÉ: Meaning "to jump" in French, sautéing involves cooking food in a small amount of hot oil. It creates a browned exterior by drawing out a plant-based food's natural sugars. This browning process not only adds color; it concentrates flavor as well. Choose a skillet that's large enough to hold your food in a single layer; piled up, it will steam rather than sauté. Heat should be at least medium. Stir often to avoid burning.

While Julia Child may have disagreed, you *can* sauté without oil. Water, broth, or another flavorful liquid can be used to create a similar effect, called "dry or water sautéing." While forgoing oil will create more of a steaming effect, the health benefits outweigh any slight compromise in color or texture.

A NOTE ON PREPPING VEGETABLES

How you cut vegetables matters. It will affect cooking times and the flavor and texture of final dish. If you aren't comfortable using a knife, consider taking a class at a local cooking store or watch a few videos on YouTube. You can sometimes use a food processor if you really don't feel comfortable with a knife, but it's worth the small time investment to learn a few basic knife

SIMMER VERSUS BOIL?

Boiling and simmering are often used interchangeably, but while they both involve hot water, they are two different cooking techniques with different purposes. Boiling is used for pasta, vegetables, and other foods that you want to cook at a high temperature and with constant motion. The bubbles will be big and rapid, and your burner will be turned to high or medium-high, depending on your stove and the amount of water and food you're cooking. Simmering is less intense, and it's used to cook foods such as root veggies or sauces more gently. The bubbles are barely visible and come to the surface one at a time every second or two. Your heat will be lower, around medium-low, and liquid is kept just below the boiling point.

skills. If you have a food processor, learn how to use it to uniformly shred and slice with ease.

To ensure foods cook at the proper rate, we provide specific instructions in each recipe. We use a few different terms to describe how to cut vegetables and other ingredients. Here's what we mean (these are not pro chef definitions, just quick explanations for busy home cooks):

CHOPPED: Cut into larger pieces, about the size of a die.

DICED: Cut into smaller pieces, about the size of a pencil eraser.

MINCED: For garlic, shallots, ginger, and anything else that you want evenly dispersed throughout a dish. Use your chef's knife to chop, chop, chop until there are no discernable pieces, or use a mini food processor (or Magic Bullet–style blender).

SLICED: Cut only in one direction. We'll usually offer further instruction, like slicing sweet potatoes into rounds or onions into half-moons.

TIP: *If you struggle to keep your vegetables from rolling all over the cutting board while you try to cut them, you're not alone. First, start with a sharp knife, which not only is safer than a dull one but will require less pressure to slice and dice. Then, use your first cut to create a flat surface for stability. So, for a sweet potato, slice off a thin piece lengthwise. Place that flat side down on the cutting board and proceed with your preparation. This works well for unruly round ingredients like carrots, potatoes, and beets.*

TIPS FOR FOOD STORAGE

There's really no sense in preparing food ahead of time or saving leftovers if you don't store it properly; otherwise, it may spoil before you can eat it. To help you make the most of your time in the kitchen—and give you more to spend elsewhere—here are some quick and easy tips for keeping food fresh.

- **Take inventory of your fridge every week before going to the grocery store.** This will also help you save money by cutting down on duplicate purchases. You'll inevitably find a rogue beet lingering in the crisper that can be used in tomorrow's lunch salad, a half-full bottle of Sriracha sauce for tonight's curry, or one last serving of Wednesday's lasagna.

- **Label and date everything.** Leftovers have an uncanny ability to go incognito in the fridge, and the freezer is a black hole for unidentified food. Black bean casserole looks like blueberry oatmeal through blurry morning eyes. (True story.) Use masking tape and a marker to write the date and name of the dish on each container, along with any pertinent reheating info. If batch cooking ahead of time, it's also useful to note quantities, such as "1 cup cooked quinoa," right on the container.

- **Keep it organized.** Instead of wasting time searching for lids to match containers, store all the lids in a bin. Every few months, sort through your collection to make sure each container has a lid. Extra lids can be recycled or replaced, while extra containers can be repurposed.

THE NO MEAT ATHLETE KITCHEN PANTRY LIST

You'll notice that our pantry list is fairly simple. That's because, without processed foods, you'll skip most aisles and buy real, whole food rather than lab-created concoctions with long ingredient lists. Here's a rundown of what fills our shopping carts each week (it varies by season, of course).

FRUIT: apples, oranges, bananas, pineapples, mangos, mixed frozen berries (for smoothies), lemons, limes

VEGETABLES: romaine or green leaf lettuce, spinach, bitter greens like dandelion or radicchio, broccoli, kale, collards, chard, celery, cucumbers, bell peppers, jalapeños, onions, carrots, tomatoes, avocados

FRESH HERBS AND AROMATICS: ginger, turmeric, garlic, basil, parsley, cilantro, scallions, red and yellow onions, shallots

STARCHY VEGETABLES: potatoes, sweet potatoes, beets, rutabagas

LEGUMES: lentils, chickpeas, beans (dry or canned)

NONWHEAT GRAINS: brown rice, quinoa (yeah, we know, it's not technically a grain), spelt or sprouted grain pasta, old-fashioned rolled oats

WHOLE WHEAT PRODUCTS (LIMITED): whole wheat or sprouted grain bread, whole wheat pasta, pitas, bagels, wraps; whole wheat flour

RAW NUTS AND SEEDS: almonds, cashews, walnuts, flaxseeds, chia seeds, Brazil nuts, pumpkin seeds (pepitas)

SPREADS, DIPS, AND PASTES: hummus, nut butters, tahini (sesame seed paste), baba ganoush, salsa, coconut butter (We sometimes make these at home, too.)

OILS (OPTIONAL, OF COURSE): olive oil, grapeseed oil, toasted sesame oil, unrefined coconut oil

VINEGARS: apple cider vinegar, balsamic vinegar, rice vinegar

PROTEIN POWDER (OPTIONAL): hemp (found in health store or online)

SOY PRODUCTS: tofu, tempeh, soy sauce (reduced-sodium tamari), or Bragg Liquid Aminos

OTHER SNACKS (LIMITED): baked tortilla chips, popcorn

MISCELLANEOUS: almond milk, coconut milk, agave nectar (as workout fuel, not an all-purpose sweetener), maple syrup, raw sugar, coffee, green tea, herbal tea (ginger, peppermint, tulsi, chamomile, etc.)

OIL-FREE
Cooking Tips

Some ingredients in a recipe can be eliminated without much impact on the texture and flavor of the final product. This is not true of oil. Omitting oil will mean less color for sautéed veggies and more sticking to the pan, especially as you learn to adjust your cooking. That said, cooking without oil is really worthwhile from a whole food–diet perspective, even if it's just part of the time. The tips that follow are a sneak peek into our oil-free cooking methods; we've integrated these tricks into the recipes in this book to preserve flavor while improving nutrition.

Note: A general rule is to use ¼ to ½ cup (60 to 120 ml) broth in place of oil for "sautéing" foods. If the liquid evaporates, feel free to add more, or use some water. In baked recipes, we specify the amount to swap.

Brown first, add liquid second. One downside of replacing oil with broth or water is that, instead of sautéing, you get more of a steaming effect and lose the color and flavor of a true sauté. To brown food without using oil, add your ingredients to a hot pan and let them sit for a minute (don't move them!) before adding the liquid to prevent burning. (To reduce the steaming effect, don't crowd the pan. Give food plenty of space in a single layer.)

Be choosy about your salt and sugar. This doesn't mean load up on them. Instead, if you choose sweet and salty ingredients with depth and substance over plain sugar or salt, you can replace much of the flavor that oil contributes. For sauces, choose dates, maple syrup, or dark brown sugar instead of plain sugar to add a caramelized flavor. Pick olives, miso, or capers for salty richness. These additional layers will add complexity and ample flavor to your final dish.

Just add booze. Typically, we use broth in place of oil when sautéing food. But instead of using a final splash of broth to release food from the pan and to scrape up the tasty bits left behind, consider using an alcoholic beverage instead. The alcohol will cook off almost entirely, and you'll be left with tons of flavor. White or red wine is a good choice, but you can also use sherry, rum (excellent in black bean dishes or those with Caribbean or Latin flavors), or bourbon (for tempeh or mushrooms).

Just keep in mind that if you wouldn't drink it, you shouldn't cook with it!

Tempted as you might be to try beer, it's not worth it! The hops will concentrate and make the dish bitter. If you're adroit at pairing beer and food, you can try it, but we've not had great luck in most cases.

Learn to deglaze.
The technique we just explained in the booze tip of using liquid to loosen any browned bits left in the pan is called deglazing. Beyond boozy liquids, consider juices (pomegranate, orange, lime, or lemon), vinegar (balsamic, apple cider, or rice), or cooking liquid from another dish. (Pasta cooking water will also add starch to thicken whatever's in the bottom of the pan.)

Lean on umami.
Fat helps develop flavor in foods, but it's not the only path to flavor town. (Sorry, did that just sound like something Guy Fieri would say?) Umami, which means "pleasant savory taste" in Japanese, is found in foods rich in glutamates—compounds that contribute a full, robust flavor to food. Meat is rich in it, but in our plant-based food pyramid, there are plenty of other umami-rich options: fermented foods, mushrooms, sea veggies, sun-dried tomatoes, tomato paste, miso, soy sauce, etc. We use plenty of these foods in our dishes.

Don't skimp on herbs and spices.
Herbs and spices are both nutritional powerhouses and flavor boosters, yet most people tend to skimp on them in dishes. They have a short shelf life (pitch dried herbs after six months to a year), so you gotta use them or lose them. Get creative and go wild with herbs and spices. It's a great way to get more comfortable in the kitchen.

Bend the rules.
Oil-free doesn't have to mean fat-free. For example, when cooking oil-free, we ditch coconut oil and use coconut milk (you can also use coconut butter or manna). We nix sesame oil but use tahini (sesame paste). Olive oil is off the list, but olives are A-OK. Nuts, avocados, and seeds are delicious and packed with healthy fats, and we think they're even more flavorful than oils.

Double up on your silicone liners and baking sheets.
Baking or roasting vegetables and tofu or tempeh without oil can yield slightly drier results, since the fat in oil creates a barrier that locks in moisture. Putting pressure on food can help it retain moisture without using oil: When roasting tempeh, tofu, or any vegetable that can lie flat on a baking sheet, place one silicone liner underneath the food and one over it (or you can use two sheets of parchment). Then, place a second baking sheet right on top. This creates gentle pressure similar to a countertop grill or panini press (but you're not going to get those grill lines) and helps to lock in moisture. It's like a lid, but rests lightly on the food and heats it from both sides.

TIME-SAVING TIP: You can get just about anything delivered these days. There are even vegan meal-kit delivery services! Save time and money on dry goods by using an online warehouse club like Thrive Market, or use Amazon Prime or Vitacost. You can even "subscribe and save" on things you buy regularly. For fresh fruits and vegetables, look for a CSA or produce home delivery option in your area. These are usually fairly affordable and are a great way to get local produce without spending your Saturday mornings at the farmers market (usually when many of us do long runs or rides).

THE LOWDOWN ON INGREDIENTS BOTH COMMON AND NOT

Here's a primer on some of the most frequently used ingredients you'll see throughout the book, including preferred brands, sourcing, and other pertinent info.

ALMOND MILK: Unless noted, assume almond milk is unsweetened and unflavored. We like the 365 brand organic unsweetened almond milk, which contains no carrageenan and has a short ingredient list.

APPLE CIDER VINEGAR: To get the maximum nutritional benefits of apple cider vinegar, it's best to use raw, unfiltered, and organic. The jury's still out on whether apple cider vinegar deserves "superfood" status, but it's rich in potassium and enzymes, promotes digestion, and its antiglycemic properties have been well researched.

ARROWROOT: We use arrowroot powder to thicken recipes and absorb moisture in breadings. It is similar to cornstarch yet superior. We prefer arrowroot's neutral flavor and more resilient nature. Arrowroot isn't starchy when undercooked, will still be effective when cooked for a long time, and can be used with acidic liquids (unlike cornstarch).

BROTH OR STOCK: For oil-free options, we just say "broth." Choose homemade or store-bought, but (we hope!) the veggie part is implied. There's no real difference between vegetable broth and vegetable stock.

CASHEWS: Unless specified, use raw, unsalted cashews. A quick soak in warm or hot water for about 10 minutes is all they need to whip up nicely in a high-speed blender. Be sure to drain them well to preserve all that creaminess.

COCONUT MILK: You can usually use light coconut milk in recipes. However, when we do call for full-fat coconut milk, it's because the extra fat is crucial to the outcome, so do not substitute it.

Though you can now find coconut milk in the refrigerated plant-based milk cooler, what you want is the stuff in cans. Most of the refrigerated versions are diluted with water (and filled with stabilizers and whiteners). They'll be fine in a cup of coffee or a bowl of granola, but they won't give the coconut flavor and richness you want in a recipe.

The Classic Unsweetened Native Forest brand (available at Whole Foods or health food stores and in bulk via Amazon) doesn't use whiteners, is organic, and comes in BPA-free cans. For oil-free recipes, it's delightfully rich and can be substituted for oil.

When recipes call for coconut milk solids only, you can reserve the liquid for smoothies. The kind with the thick, white cream on top is what you want in our Vegan-Edge Waffles (page 51).

COCONUT OIL: Coconut oil is incredibly versatile in plant-based cooking, but we use it sparingly. We recommend unrefined or virgin coconut oil. (Refined coconut oil is best used for frying, which is not a cooking technique we use in this book!) Coconut oil is solid at room temperature and melts at 76°F (24°C). In winter, you may have to chisel off a chunk for your recipes; in summer, it'll pour with ease. Unless noted in baked goods, you can use melted or solid coconut oil.

FLOUR: The recipes in this book always use whole wheat flour. You want the fiber and, especially, the protein and nutrients from the whole grain. It tends to be coarser than all-purpose flour, so for baked goods, we often use whole wheat pastry flour, which is finely ground but nutritionally the same as regular whole wheat flour.

HERBS AND SPICES: Fresh is implied, unless noted. (Spoiler alert: You always want fresh herbs to garnish a dish. Otherwise, you can usually swap them in recipes.) If you're using dried in place of fresh, use one third of the amount. Fresh herbs typically should be added at the end of cooking, while dried can be added at the beginning. Always crush or rub dried herbs before adding them to release their fragrance and flavor. Dried herbs lose their potency quickly, so buy only what you can use within a few months.

KALE: It's your choice on varieties. You can use curly or flat-leafed kale. We like to save stems for smoothies.

MATCHA: Matcha is dried, finely ground green tea leaves that are specifically cultivated to be ground up and consumed (versus steeped and strained). There are two grades: ceremonial and culinary. For all recipes, the latter is fine (and is much cheaper). Add it to smoothies, oatmeal, and baked goods for a dose of antioxidants (including heart-supporting polyphenols).

MISO PASTE: Miso is fermented soybean paste. It's packed with probiotics and contributes a salty, savory note to dishes. You'll find it in the refrigerated section of your supermarket (often with the tofu and vegan meat substitutes) divided by color.

Red miso (akamiso) is aged longer and has a bolder, richer flavor. It's great for adding meaty, robust flavor to soups and many other dishes. White miso (shiromiso) is mild and sweet, and it can be made with chickpeas, too. We use the Miso Master brand, which is handcrafted just outside Asheville using traditional Japanese methods.

Worth noting:

- We advise against using one when the other is called for (think: sweet versus deep, rich flavors); the results will not be comparable. Though miso is pricey, it lasts for up to a year in the fridge, so it's not something you'll have to throw away in a week if you only need a spoonful.

- Never boil miso. It will kill the beneficial bacteria. Whisk it in at the end of cooking after your food has stopping boiling.

- Avoid varieties with the word "dashi" or "bonito" on the package; this means it contains fish.

NUTRITIONAL YEAST: These yellow flakes are commonly used to boost umami and "cheesy" flavor in plant-based recipes. A form of inert yeast, nutritional yeast contains 8 grams of protein and 4 grams of fiber per 1½ tablespoon serving. Choose varieties that are fortified with B vitamins, such as Red Star or Bragg. Find it in the bulk section of your supermarket or in shaker-top containers in the herbs and spices aisle.

SALT AND PEPPER: Unless noted, use salt and pepper to taste in most dishes, usually waiting until the end to add salt to a dish so as to limit its use. We primarily use freshly ground black pepper and fine Celtic sea salt. For "finishing" a dish, you can choose a high-quality coarse or flaky salt, such as Maldon.

SEA VEGETABLES: These are valuable sources of nutrition (especially minerals), so we don't want to call them "weeds"! Some people don't care for the fishy taste of many sea veggies, so we've made them optional in most cases.

Agar: We use agar as a thickening agent in our No-Bake Mocha Cheesecake (page 258). Made from algae, these clear flakes (it also comes in block form) are traditionally used to thicken Japanese jelly desserts. You can find it in the Asian aisle of most supermarkets, and at Japanese grocers it may be called *kanten*. Get creative with your agar, but don't use it with citrus, as the acid will prevent it from setting properly.

Dulse: Dulse is a reddish brown sea vegetable that's grown in the northern Atlantic and Pacific. When lightly pan-fried (with or without oil), it takes on the texture of bacon, with (arguably) a similar taste. You can use it crumbled on our Lifesaving Bowl (page 88), atop stir-fries, or in sandwiches. It provides iron, calcium, magnesium and potassium, among other vitamins and minerals.

Kombu: We like to add a 1-inch (2.5 cm) square of this sea veggie to our beans as they cook to add depth of flavor and increase digestibility. Kombu is high in iodine and contains iron and calcium.

Nori: If you've eaten sushi, you've had nori, aka laver. It's the wrapper used in most rolls. Nori contains plenty of minerals, and the toasted sheets add crunch when crumbled over rice or steamed veggies. The single packs of nori make a fun snack, too. Note that pretoasted varieties are often coated in sesame or vegetable oil, so avoid those if you're oil-free.

Wakame: This is the sea vegetable you typically see floating in your miso soup. It does have a slightly fishy taste, so if that's a turnoff, feel free to omit it. It's a good source of magnesium and adds quite a bit of flavor as well as a chewy texture.

SOY: To soy or not to soy? This is a hot topic in the plant-based world. We're fine with it in whole food (edamame) or fermented (tempeh, miso) form. It's ubiquitous in vegan food, so we get plenty of it. But we aim to eat a diverse diet, so while we like soy, we often use other beans or choose nut milk over soy milk to ensure plenty of variety.

SOY SAUCE: We sometimes use this general term to cover many bases. We usually choose either Bragg Liquid Aminos or organic reduced-sodium tamari, which is also gluten-free. You can sub in coconut aminos, regular soy sauce, or another salty condiment. We recommend reduced-sodium, regardless of your choice.

SWEETENERS: Use these sparingly and try to keep them as natural and unrefined as possible. When we say "sugar," we mean some kind of less-refined granulated sugar: demerara, Sucanat, turbinado, or evaporated cane juice (soon to be called just "sugar"). When we say "sweetener," you can expand that to include maple syrup, agave, brown rice syrup, or anything else. We note when a specific sweetener is needed.

Our recipes are generally not very sweet, and you'll probably find that the longer you eat a whole food, plant-based diet, the less you'll crave sweets. Feel free to adjust the sweetness to your taste, but keep in mind that sugar, no matter how unrefined, is still sugar, and when it's not part of whole fruit or used to fuel a workout, it's not a health food. We note anytime a precise measurement cannot be adjusted.

TEMPEH: Tempeh is a fermented, minimally processed legume product that you can find in most grocery stores these days. Though it's usually made from soy, it can also be made from any combination of legumes and grains. The beneficial bacteria in tempeh break down the legumes so they are more easily digested. We're lucky to have Smiling Hara Tempeh here in Asheville,

ON CREATIVITY
How to Successfully Hack a Recipe (If That's Your Thing)

I f you're the kind of person who likes to buy cookbooks but not follow the recipes to a T, we understand. We encourage you to get creative with these recipes and truly make them your own. Our testers did, usually with great success.

But there are a few things you should keep in mind before you start playing Iron Chef with these (or any) recipes. We share these tips not because it's our way or the highway, but because we know that food matters. We don't want you to waste time, money, and energy on a doctored recipe only to have it be a flop!

Take inventory. The shorter the ingredient list, the more crucial the individual components are. For example, take our Tahini Green Beans (page 158) and Breakfast Hummus (page 56), which both contain tahini. In the hummus, it's one of over a dozen ingredients. There are only five main ingredients in the green beans, and tahini is one of them (and in the recipe title!). Omitting it or changing the

tahini in the green beans dish will have more of an impact. Unless you feel pretty confident in your cooking, don't mess with an ingredient when it'll have a major impact. (Or do, but be ready for the outcome.)

Do sweat the small stuff. Oftentimes, it's the pinches, teaspoons, and dashes of ingredients that matter most in recipes: the salt to bring out the sweetness in cookies, the acid to provide contrast to a sauce, or the tamari to add umami to a stir-fry. If you're going to swap one of the seasonings, it may impact the final result. Though counterintuitive, it's usually less risky to swap out major ingredients (see the next tip for more on that) than it is to mess with the small stuff.

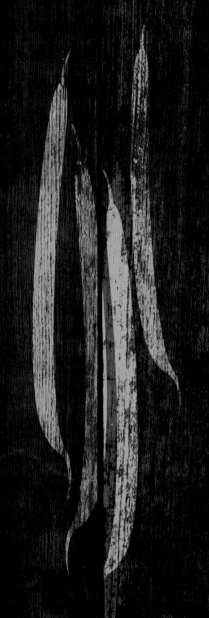

Apples to apples—and apples to pears.
You have carte blanche to use pinto beans instead
of black beans, broccoli instead of cauliflower, or
hemp milk instead of almond milk—and any other
swap of ingredients that seems similar. When
ingredients are so alike, there's little risk of spoiling
the recipe.

Walk before you run. If you're new to cooking, it's best to stick with the recipes as they're
written. Once you're fairly comfortable in the
kitchen, however, feel free to start improvising—
making "mistakes" is how you get better!

Start with the blueprints. Throughout the
book, we have labeled several recipes "Blueprints."
These simple meals provide the foundation for a
foolproof dish that you can riff upon as desired. If
you're new to "cooking outside the lines," these are
a great place to start, as we've designed them to be
incredibly forgiving.

KEY TO ICONS AND ABBREVIATIONS

FF: Fast food. On days you need to eat, like, now, look for this icon, which will mark any recipe that's ready start to finish in 30 minutes or less. We also use this icon for tips to get food on the table faster.

SF: Slow food. We give you the heads-up if something requires an hour or more of rest and prep time, such as the No-Bake Mocha Cheesecake (page 258) or Slow-Cooker Brown Rice Porridge (page 46).

SC: Slow cooker. We love the slow cooker, but we know you need a heads-up if something's gonna take all day to cook. You'll see this in our Better than Bone Broth (page 210) and Slow-Cooker Refried Beans (page 174), for example.

CL: Carbo loading. For those days when you need to top off your glycogen stores, we've

noted the recipes that are good for "carbo loading."

GF/GFO: Gluten-free/gluten-free option. We highlight the recipes that are naturally gluten-free or can easily become gluten-free. Of course, if you have a gluten intolerance or celiac disease, please read all labels carefully to avoid risk of cross-contamination. We also offer tips to cut the gluten when possible.

OF/OFO: Oil-free/oil-free option. See pages 30–31 for more on oil-free cooking.

XS: Soy-free. Because many people prefer to avoid soy, we call out recipes that are soy-free. For recipes that call for "reduced-sodium tamari" simply swap in coconut aminos or another soy-free salty condiment.

so that's what we use. Their tempeh (including some 100 percent soy-free varieties made from black beans or other legumes) is available across the Southeast and online. If you can't find Smiling Hara or one of the other artisan tempehs across the United States, choose organic tempeh to ensure that the soybeans are non-GMO.

To remove the bitter taste tempeh often has, cube it or pierce the block all over with

a fork and then steam it for 10 minutes over 1 inch (2.5 cm) of water before using it in a recipe.

TOFU: Unless noted, we suggest using organic, extra-firm tofu. Choose a sprouted variety if available. In the eastern United States, Twin Oaks is a good choice. It's made in Virginia by a small co-op. Their herbed tofu is delicious enough to slice raw, sprinkle with salt and pepper, and eat on a sandwich.

TOMATOES: Look for jars or brands that do not use BPA in their can lining, such as Muir Glen. Choosing "no salt added" varieties allows you to control the sodium content yourself, but because they're not always easy to find, our recipes assume you're using regular, salted canned tomatoes. In season, feel free to use fresh tomatoes. (Avoid pureeing whole fresh tomatoes, as the seeds add bitterness. Crush or chop them instead.)

UMEBOSHI PASTE: An umami-rich paste made from pickled, salted sour plums. The color comes from red shiso leaves. Ume plums are good for digestion, and the Japanese use them to help nausea (and hangovers). They are also thought to promote stamina and were a part of the samurais' field rations! The salty-sour taste helps combat dry mouth on long runs. You can find them in the Asian aisle of most grocery stores.

WHITE BEANS: You can use cannellini (white kidney) or navy beans when we don't specify the type of white bean in a recipe.

SOME FINAL NOTES

Choosing Organic. Of course it's a good idea to eat organic and local whenever possible, but we understand it's a personal choice based on geography, budget, and other resources. As such, we encourage you to prioritize buying organic produce that is on the Environmental Working Group's "Dirty Dozen" list (available at ewg.org/foodnews/dirty_dozen_list.php or via their "Dirty Dozen" app).

It's All Vegan! This is a 100 percent plant-based cookbook, so we omit the word "vegan" where it would be superfluous. So for example, we say "chocolate chips," not "*vegan* chocolate chips," even though we mean the latter.

Timing Is Relative. Cooking is like running; everyone will have a pace that feels comfortable to them. We did our best to account for this in our prep times, but you may find that your own timing is a bit faster or slower.

SERVINGS AND NUTRITION INFO

We have included serving info for each recipe as a whole, as we know that every reader will divide the dish differently and in varying portion sizes. An Ironman in training may take down a whole pan of Baked Deep-Dish Apple Pancake (page 48) at breakfast the day after an event, while a power yogi may be satisfied with just a slice.

We opted against including nutrition info for every recipe, as these whole-food, plant-based recipes are inherently healthy and appropriate even for those on a reduced-calorie diet. However, if you do count calories or track your macros, you can find the nutrition facts for every recipe in this book at nomeatathlete.com /nutrition-info.

We did include the nutrition info for Chapter 7, as fueling is a time when athletes pay close attention to calorie and macronutrient composition. To determine nutrition facts for those recipes, we used the recipe feature at the MyFitnessPal website, double-checking each ingredient and quantity. Nutrition info was calculated using the basic recipe (not any variations or optional ingredients) and is meant to provide general guidance. We include separate fat and calorie info for oil-free versions in relevant recipes. We have omitted cholesterol from the nutrition info, because every recipe is cholesterol-free: Cholesterol is only present in animal products!

OIL-FREE COOKING OPTIONS

As we both eat differently when it comes to oil, we put a lot of thought into whether or not to include it in the recipes in this book. And we decided . . . not to decide. We did both! As we mentioned in Chapter 1, every recipe in this book, if not oil-free as is, includes an oil-free cooking option.

To make the oil-free version of any dish that includes oil, note the "OF" substitution next to oil in the ingredient list of that recipe. In some cases it will simply say "OF: omit," and in these cases you can just proceed with the recipe as written, omitting the oil when it's mentioned in the recipe instructions. In other cases, we'll call for the oil to be replaced with water, broth, nut butter, or another substitute ingredient, and when we do, we'll let you know what amount to use if it's different from the amount of oil called for, and provide any specific instructions that are required as the recipe proceeds.

The transition to an oil-free, plant-based diet is a big one indeed, and we hope that if it's something that interests you, our decision to include oil-free versions of every recipe will make it easy for you to experiment.

Part Two

Recipes
&
Meal Plans

Chapter 3

MORNING MEALS TO MOTIVATE & POWER YOUR DAY

I n his book *The Blue Zones*, author and researcher Dan Buettner takes a look at the pockets of societies around the world that produce the largest number of centenarians (people who are 100 years old or older) per capita. The results are not only fascinating, but they affirm the benefits of a plant-based diet—and they have more than a few things to say about the way we should eat breakfast.

You know that old "breakfast is the most important meal of the day" maxim that new-school diets have taken pride in ignoring? Well, it's back. The longest-lived people on earth typically eat very large breakfasts, medium-size lunches, and relatively small dinners. Of course, this all falls apart if your breakfast is loaded with added sugar and other processed carbohydrates, so you'll note that our breakfasts are big on flavor and portion size but short on sugar and refined grains.

Beans make a frequent appearance at the breakfast tables of Blue Zones families. We know what you're thinking: *Beans for breakfast?* Actually, it's not as hard (or strange) as it seems. In this section we've got recipes for Breakfast Hummus (based on chickpeas and used in The Daily Grinder sandwich and our Rise & Shine Salad), Chickpea Quiche, two ways to do Breakfast Tofu, and several burrito recipes that include either beans or tofu. Of course, there are a few treatlike morning meals included, more for fueling a long mid-morning workout or simply to enjoy, but even these are designed to provide sustained energy rather than a sugar rush.

If we're trying to eat like the world's longest-lived people, though, there's one aspect in which we typically fall short by virtue of the culture in which we live . . . and it's that most of us eat breakfast on the go. Ideally, we'd all take our time to savor our breakfast seated at a table, but our modern, Western world is set up in such a way that there's not a whole lot of time between when the sun rises and when we've got to be at work or school. But eating in the car, at our desk, or while we're getting ready to leave the house doesn't have to mean eating junk food. To this end, we've developed many of our or breakfast recipes so that they're easy to eat on the move or take with you to work. On days when you've got some space in your morning, we encourage you to enjoy these breakfasts at the table, but trust us—we know what it's like to try to fit a workout, a shower, and a commute into your morning, and a portable breakfast is a huge help on busy days.

SAVORY OATMEAL

MAKES: 2 bowls // **TIME:** 15 minutes

Oatmeal is an incredibly popular breakfast among athletes and health foodies, but even if you vary the toppings, it's easy to get bored with the same sweet flavors every morning. But who said oatmeal has to be sweet? This savory recipe lends itself well to customization, so you can adapt it to suit your palate and vary it when you want something new.

1 cup (95 g) GF old-fashioned rolled oats

1 carrot or small beet, peeled and shredded

1½ cups (360 ml) water

1 cup (15 g) stemmed and chopped kale or (30 g) chopped spinach

¼ cup (60 g) salsa or marinara sauce (such as Weeknight Marinara, page 81)

2 tablespoons nutritional yeast

½ avocado, chopped

2 tablespoons roasted pumpkin seeds

Smoked paprika and/or crushed red pepper, optional

Salt and black pepper

1 Combine the oats and carrot in a small saucepan over medium heat. Add the water. (Use more or less to achieve the consistency you prefer; 1½ cups/360 ml water yields a fairly thick oatmeal.)

2 Heat until simmering, then cook, stirring often, until everything is tender, about 5 minutes.

3 Stir in the kale, salsa, and nutritional yeast.

4 Pour into a bowl and top with the avocado and pumpkin seeds. Sprinkle with smoked paprika and crushed red pepper, if using. Season with salt and pepper to taste, and serve.

Variation: Swap in different flavors of salsas or pasta sauces to turn this into a whole new dish.

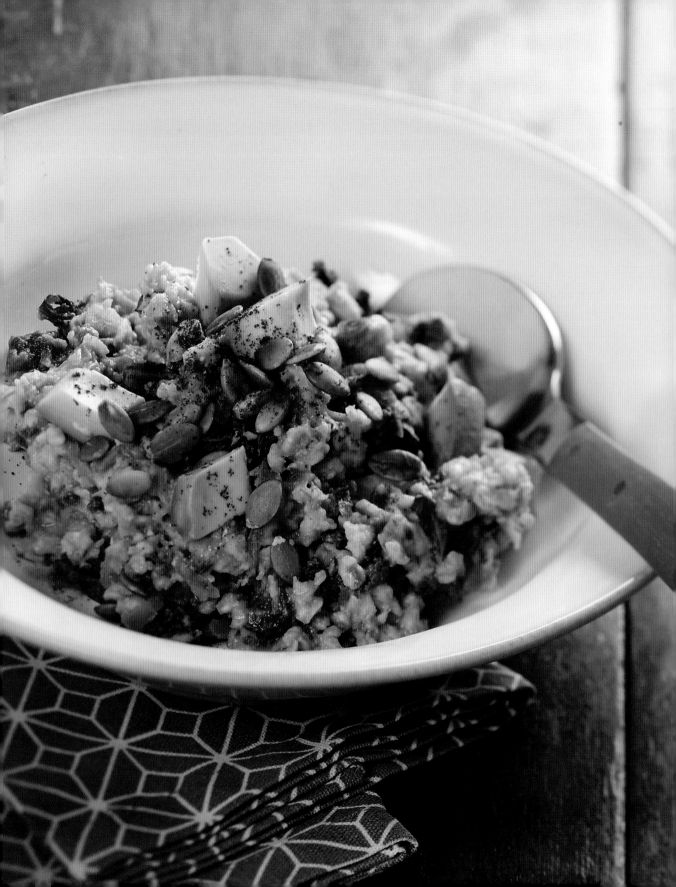

SLOW-COOKER BROWN RICE PORRIDGE

MAKES: 2 bowls // **TIME:** 15 minutes to prep, 8 hours to cook

This slow-cooker rice porridge is based on the Korean staple *juk,* which comes in dozens of variations. This dish is designed to be a make-ahead breakfast that cooks while you sleep, then stays warm until you're ready to eat. You can also eat it as a light dinner or snack.

1 carrot, diced

2 garlic cloves, minced

1 teaspoon toasted sesame oil (OF: 1 teaspoon tahini mixed with ¼ cup/60 ml broth)

1 cup (180 g) short-grain brown rice

4 cups (960 ml) vegetable broth

1½ cups (360 ml) water

Reduced-sodium, GF tamari or red miso

2 scallions, white and light green parts, sliced

1 sheet nori, snipped or crumbled into bite-size pieces

Toasted sesame seeds

1 If your slow cooker has a sauté setting, turn it to high (if not, do the first two steps in a saucepan on the stove). Add the carrot, garlic, and sesame oil. Cook, stirring often, until the carrot starts to soften, about 5 minutes.

2 Stir in the rice. Cook for 5 minutes.

3 Add the broth and water. Turn the slow cooker to low, cover, set for 8 hours, and go to bed!

4 In the morning, stir the porridge and season with tamari to taste. Garnish with scallions, nori, and sesame seeds and serve.

SLOW-COOKER COCONUT-MATCHA BROWN RICE

MAKES: 2 bowls // **TIME:** 5 minutes to prep, 8 hours to cook

Matcha (green tea powder) offers bright color as well as a boost of energy and antioxidants to this sweet slow-cooked porridge. Since the matcha is cooked right into the dish, you can get the benefits of green tea without having to take the time to brew a cup in the morning. It's really good with cold coconut milk poured over top, too.

1 Turn your slow cooker to low. Add the coconut milk, rice, matcha, and vanilla and stir to combine. Add the water, cover, and set for 8 hours.

2 In the morning, stir the porridge and add maple syrup to taste. Garnish with coconut, pistachios, and cardamom and serve.

1 cup (240 ml) light coconut milk

1 cup (180 g) short-grain brown rice

1 tablespoon matcha powder

¼ teaspoon vanilla extract

5 cups (1.2 L) water

Maple syrup or other sweetener

Unsweetened shredded coconut

Chopped unsalted pistachios

Ground cardamom

OFO XS CL

BAKED DEEP-DISH APPLE PANCAKE

MAKES: one 8- to 9-inch (20 to 23 cm) pancake; serves 6 to 8
TIME: 10 minutes to prep, 30 to 35 minutes to bake

This baked pancake tastes like dessert, but it's substantial and healthy enough to serve as breakfast. Bonus: The leftovers can be wrapped in parchment and eaten midway through a workout. This is one of the sweetest recipes in the book, so if your apples are on the sweeter side, you might want to scale back on sugar and maple syrup.

4 tart apples (such as Gala, Honeycrisp, or Granny Smith), peeled, cored, and thinly sliced

¼ cup (30 g) chopped walnuts or pecans, optional

1 teaspoon ground cinnamon

1½ cups (225 g) whole wheat flour

2 teaspoons baking powder

¼ teaspoon plus ⅛ teaspoon salt

1 cup (240 ml) light or full-fat coconut milk

2 tablespoons maple syrup

1 tablespoon plus 1 teaspoon fresh lemon juice

1 teaspoon vanilla extract

¼ cup (35 g) unpacked dark brown sugar or coconut sugar

1 tablespoon coconut oil (OF: omit)

1 Preheat the oven to 375°F (190°C). Place a deep cast-iron skillet over medium heat. Once it's warm, add the apples, ½ teaspoon cinnamon, and walnuts, if using, in a single layer. Let the apples cook while you prepare the batter.

2 Combine the flour, baking powder, ¼ teaspoon salt, and remaining ½ teaspoon cinnamon in a medium bowl. In a separate bowl, stir the coconut milk, maple syrup, 1 tablespoon lemon juice, and vanilla together, then pour into the dry ingredients and whisk until just combined.

3 Sprinkle the sugar, remaining 1 teaspoon lemon juice, and remaining ⅛ teaspoon salt over the apples. Remove from the heat, and add the coconut oil to the pan, focusing on the perimeter of the apples. (OF: Be sure to use a well-seasoned pan.)

4 Pour the batter on top and bake for 30 to 35 minutes, until the pancake is cooked through and golden brown. Slice into wedges, scoop onto plates, and serve.

ALMOND BUTTER–BANANA PANCAKES OR WAFFLES

MAKES: 4 waffles or 8 pancakes // **TIME:** 5 minutes to prep, 25 minutes to cook

Aside from being hearty pre-workout or take-along meals, pancakes and waffles make for convenient kid-friendly breakfasts. We like to make them ahead of time and freeze them, reheating in the toaster each morning and serving with fruit. These are quite substantial and mildly sweet, which makes kids (and parents!) happy. Sugar is optional in this recipe; use it only if you won't be eating yours with syrup or jam. These get super crispy on the outside thanks to the almond meal but stay quite moist and tender on the inside.

1 Preheat a griddle over medium-high heat (or preheat a waffle iron).

2 Combine the almond milk, banana, almond butter, chia seeds, sugar (if using), and vanilla in a blender. Puree until smooth. (For pancakes, add ¼ cup/60 ml water.)

3 Combine the flour, almond meal, baking powder, cinnamon, and salt in a medium bowl. Pour the wet ingredients into the dry and fold until just combined.

For waffles: Grease your waffle iron. Add ½ cup (120 ml) batter to the center of your iron. Cook for about 6 minutes, or until cooked through. Repeat with remaining batter and serve.

For pancakes: Grease the griddle. Add ¼ cup (60 ml) batter and cook until bubbles have formed and popped (about 2 minutes); flip and cook another 2 to 3 minutes, until the center is cooked. Repeat with the remaining batter and serve.

NOTE: *Don't be alarmed if these look darker than your usual pancakes or waffles. They will be dark brown from the banana. Shades of brown are normal—just don't let them turn black.*

OF: *Truly oil-free waffles or pancakes are tricky if your waffle iron or pan isn't well seasoned or nonstick. (Most aren't.) But that doesn't mean you have to miss out. Pour the batter into a 9-inch (23 cm) cast-iron skillet or silicone cake pan. Bake at 375°F (190°C) for 35 to 40 minutes, until a toothpick inserted in the center comes out clean.*

1 cup (240 ml) almond milk

1 ripe banana

2 tablespoons almond butter

2 tablespoons chia seeds

2 tablespoons sugar, optional

½ teaspoon vanilla extract

¾ cup (90 g) whole wheat pastry flour

½ cup (55 g) almond meal or additional pastry flour

2 teaspoons baking powder

¼ teaspoon ground cinnamon

⅛ teaspoon salt

Oil, for greasing (OF: See below)

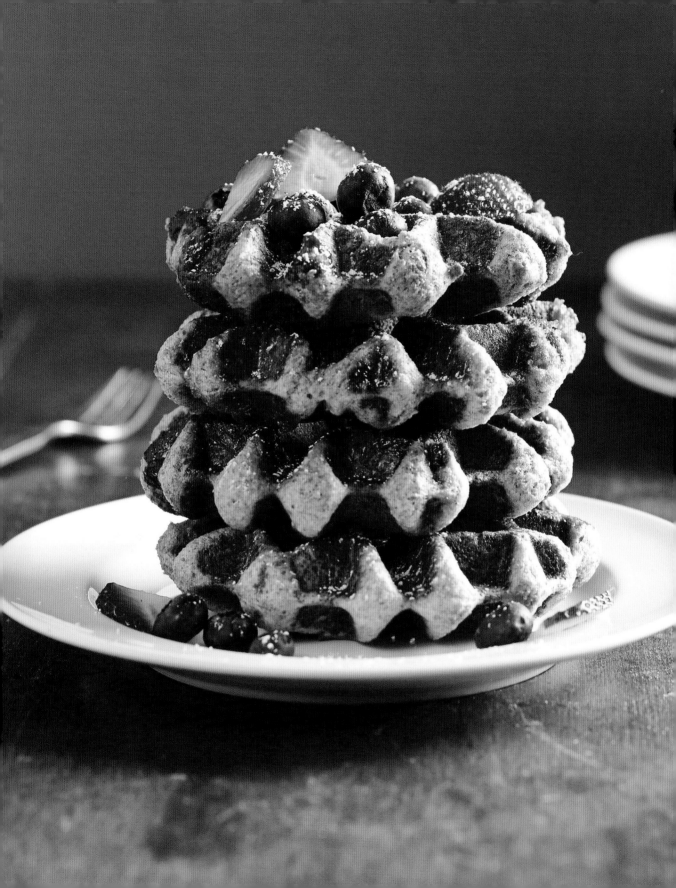

VEGAN-EDGE WAFFLES

MAKES: 12 waffles // **TIME:** 15 minutes to prepare, 2 hours to rise and bake

These waffles are simple yet decadent. The crushed sugar cubes create pockets of brown sugar goodness on the inside and a caramelized glaze on parts of the outside. You can slice them in half horizontally and slather with salted nut butter for a mid-workout sandwich. The name of these waffles gives a nod to the movie *Scott Pilgrim vs. the World* (there's a character who gets an "edge" from plant-based eating) and kinda rhymes with the traditional name for these Belgian waffles, Liège, which are popular in Europe at cyclo-cross races. These are much lighter than the originals: They are oil-free, use far less sugar, and are made with whole wheat flour. Our recipe is based on a non-vegan version, from the blog *Smitten Kitchen*.

1 In a small saucepan set over medium, heat the almond milk until it is just warmer than your skin temperature. Transfer to a large bowl and whisk in the brown sugar and yeast. Set aside for 5 minutes.

2 Scrape the solids from the coconut milk into a small bowl. Pour in the liquid and whisk until fluffy. Stir in the vanilla. Fold the coconut cream into the almond milk mixture.

3 Whisk in 2 cups (240 g) of the flour and the salt. Add another 1½ cups (180 g) flour, switching to a wooden spoon when the dough starts to come together. The dough will be sticky. Cover and set in a warm, moist place to rise for an hour.

4 Stir in the sugar cubes and the remaining ½ cup (60 g) flour. The dough will be slightly sticky but still workable. (At this point, you can refrigerate the dough overnight.)

5 Preheat and grease a Belgian waffle iron. Divide the dough evenly into 12 balls. Drop one dough ball onto the iron and close it firmly. Cook for about 6 minutes, or until golden brown. (These waffles are thick, so break open your first one to see whether it's fully cooked, as waffle irons vary. If it is not, simply keep cooking it.)

6 Repeat with the remaining dough, and serve. (Waffles can be wrapped individually in parchment paper and refrigerated in an airtight container for up to 3 days or frozen for up to 3 months. To reheat, toast in a 300°F/150°C oven until warmed through and crispy on the outside.)

¾ cup (180 ml) almond milk

¼ cup (55 g) packed dark brown or raw sugar

One ¼-ounce (7 g) packet active dry yeast

One 13.5-ounce (400 ml) can full-fat coconut milk

1½ teaspoons vanilla extract

4 cups (480 g) whole wheat pastry flour

1 teaspoon salt

½ cup (110 g) raw sugar cubes, crushed roughly into quarters with a mortar and pestle

Oil, for greasing (OF: See page 49 for baking directions if your waffle iron isn't truly nonstick.)

NUT BUTTER & JELLY BREAKFAST COOKIES

MAKES: 24 cookies // **TIME:** 10 minutes to prep, 20 minutes to bake

These kid-friendly breakfast cookies were inspired by a recipe from vegan cookbook author Joni Marie Newman. But while the original used white flour, traditional jam, and peanut butter, our healthier version has whole wheat flour, less sugar, and whole fruit. Take some with you on a run. If you use crunchy nut butter, or if your nut butter is on the drier or thicker side, you should use about ¼ cup (30 g) less flour.

¾ cup (190 g) nut butter (we like a combo of almond butter and cashew butter)

½ cup (75 g) berries or 1 small banana, mashed with a fork

¼ cup plus 2 tablespoons (120 g) fruit preserves

1 to 1¼ cups (150 to 190 g) whole wheat flour

¾ teaspoon baking powder

⅛ teaspoon salt

① Preheat the oven to 350°F (180°C). Line two baking sheets with parchment paper.

② Add the nut butter, berries, and preserves to a food processor. Pulse until thoroughly combined. Add 1 cup (150 g) of the flour, the baking powder, and salt, continuing to pulse until combined. Add additional flour, as needed, until a thick dough forms. The dough should be smooth and glossy (almost greasy), with no visible flour. If needed, transfer to a bowl and knead the dough until the flour is fully incorporated.

③ Divide the dough into 12 pieces, roll each piece into a ball, then flatten into a cookie shape; add the traditional peanut butter cookie hashmarks with a fork if desired.

④ Bake for 17 to 20 minutes, until the tops are golden brown. Allow to cool completely on the baking sheet before serving. (Cookies can be stored at room temperature in an airtight container for up to 5 days.)

NOTE: *Baking powder has an expiration date, and its shelf life is shorter than you might think. The label says it lasts about 18 months, but once opened, it's only useful for about 6 months. Old baking powder won't allow your dough or batter to rise, so you'll end up with dense, flat baked goods. If you can't remember when you last bought baking powder or you only bake once a year or so, pitch it. You can test to see if yours is still working by mixing ¼ teaspoon baking powder with ½ cup (120 ml) hot water (tap is fine). If it bubbles, it's still good. If not, buy more before baking. We use aluminum-free baking powder for both health and taste. Baking powder with aluminum can give your food a slightly metallic, tinny taste.*

SAVORY ROSEMARY–BLACK PEPPER SCONES

MAKES: 8 scones // **TIME:** 10 minutes to prep, 20 minutes to cook

Think of these scones as a quicker, healthier version of biscuits. You can serve them with a tofu scramble and Miso Gravy (page 231) on weekends, or split in half and top with avocado and nutritional yeast for a quick breakfast. For dinner, serve them with French Onion Stew with Mushrooms (page 126), atop Pasta Marinara (page 81), or under Harissa Baked Tofu (page 71). Swap in different herbs to customize them; try scallion-dill or tarragon–lemon zest, for example. In this recipe, coconut oil replaces butter or shortening, so you want it to be semisolid or solid. If yours is soft, measure it out, then freeze for about 10 minutes before using.

1 Preheat the oven to 475°F (245°C). Lightly grease a baking sheet (or use parchment paper).

2 Mix the flour, oats, rosemary, baking powder, pepper, and salt in a medium bowl. Add the coconut oil and—using a pastry cutter, two forks, or your fingers—mix until well combined. Add the almond milk and lemon juice and mix with a fork until it forms a shaggy ball of dough; do not overmix.

3 Split the dough into two balls. Spread one ball of dough into a circle on one end of the sheet. It should be 1 inch (2.5 cm) thick. Repeat on the other side. Use a knife to cut each circle into 4 wedges.

4 Bake for 20 minutes, or until a toothpick inserted in the middle comes out clean and the scones are golden brown. Serve warm. (Toast any leftovers before serving.)

1 cup (150 g) whole wheat flour

¾ cup (60 g) old-fashioned rolled oats

2 tablespoons minced fresh rosemary

½ teaspoon baking powder

½ teaspoon freshly ground black pepper

½ teaspoon salt

3 tablespoons solid coconut oil (OF: 3 tablespoons pureed white beans or tahini)

¾ cup (180 ml) almond milk

1 tablespoon fresh lemon juice

BLUEBERRY SCONES

MAKES: 8 scones // **TIME:** 10 minutes to prep, 20 minutes to cook

Serve these sweet breakfast scones as is or with a smear of jam. The variations are endless: Substitute dried currants or cranberries, or use fresh strawberries or raspberries with plenty of lemon zest in place of the blueberries. In this recipe, coconut oil or coconut butter replaces butter or shortening, so you want it to be semisolid or solid. If yours is soft, measure it out, then freeze for about 10 minutes before using.

1 cup (150 g) whole wheat flour

¾ cup (60 g) old-fashioned rolled oats

½ teaspoon baking powder

½ teaspoon salt

1 cup (150 g) blueberries, thawed and drained if frozen

3 tablespoons solid coconut oil (OF: 3 tablespoons cold coconut butter)

¾ cup (180 ml) almond milk

1 tablespoon fresh lemon juice

2 teaspoons raw or granulated sugar

1 Preheat the oven to 475°F (245°C). Lightly grease a baking sheet (or use parchment paper).

2 Mix the flour, oats, baking powder, and salt in a medium bowl. Add the coconut oil and—using a pastry cutter, two forks, or your fingers—mix until well combined. Fold in the blueberries. Add the almond milk and lemon juice and mix with a fork until it forms a shaggy ball of dough; do not overmix.

3 Split the dough into two balls. Spread one ball of dough into a circle on one end of the sheet. It should be 1 inch (2.5 cm) thick. Repeat on the other side. Sprinkle 1 teaspoon of sugar over each circle. Use a knife to cut each circle into 4 wedges.

4 Bake for 20 minutes, or until a toothpick inserted in the middle comes out clean and the scones are golden brown. Serve warm. (Toast any leftovers before serving.)

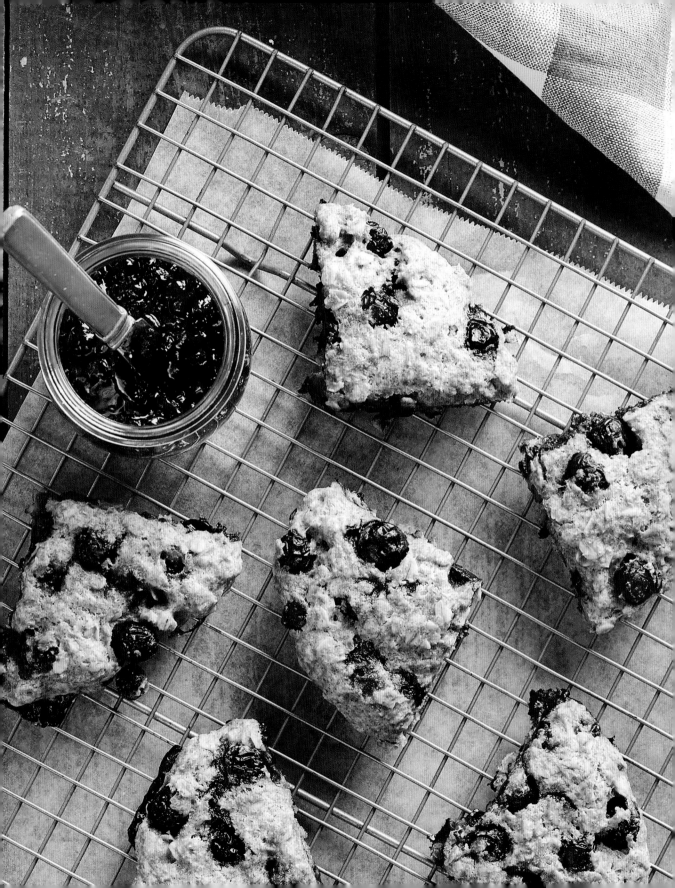

TOAST, ELEVATED

Toast is a portable, easy breakfast. Whole wheat bread has plenty of protein to power you through to lunchtime, and we choose sprouted or sourdough so it's easier to digest. Here are some of our favorite takes on toast, including some new twists on the ever-popular avocado variety and a breakfast version of hummus with flavors similar to those of a tofu scramble.

1 tablespoon olive oil (OF:
¼ cup/60 ml broth)

1 yellow onion, diced

1 garlic clove, minced

1 teaspoon ground cumin

1 teaspoon smoked paprika

½ teaspoon curry powder

½ teaspoon ground turmeric

¼ teaspoon black pepper, plus more
to taste

1 sprig thyme

2 cups (480 ml) water

1 cup (200 g) dried chickpeas,
soaked overnight, drained,
and rinsed

½ cup (30 g) nutritional yeast

2 tablespoons tahini, GF if
necessary

1 tablespoon reduced-sodium
tamari or red miso,
GF if necessary

Salt

Toast, GF if necessary, for serving

BREAKFAST HUMMUS ON TOAST

SERVES: 8 to 12 // Makes: about 3 cups (675 g) hummus
TIME: 1 hour

1 Heat a medium saucepan over medium heat, then add the oil. Add the onion and sauté, stirring often, until softened, about 5 minutes. Add the garlic, cumin, paprika, curry powder, turmeric, ¼ teaspoon pepper, and thyme and cook 2 minutes longer.

2 Add the water and chickpeas. Increase the heat to high, bring to a boil, then reduce to medium-low and cook, covered, until tender, about 45 minutes.

3 Drain the chickpeas, reserving the cooking water. Transfer the chickpeas to a food processor along with the nutritional yeast, tahini, and tamari. Pulse to combine, then puree until smooth, adding the cooking liquid 1 tablespoon at a time to achieve the desired consistency. (The hummus will thicken slightly as it cools.)

4 Season with salt and pepper to taste, and serve on toast. (The hummus can be refrigerated for up to 5 days.)

FF: *Use two 15-ounce (425 g) cans chickpeas, drained, instead of cooking dried ones (and omit the water). Sauté the onion and spices as directed, then add that mixture to the blender with the chickpeas and proceed with the recipe. You may want to add some water (up to ½ cup/120 ml), to achieve the desired consistency.*

PAN CON TOMATE

MAKES: 2 slices // **TIME:** 10 minutes

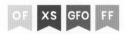

Rub each slice of toast with a garlic clove half and half a Roma tomato. Sprinkle with salt and, if desired, nutritional yeast.

NOTE: *The rough texture of the bread sort of melts the garlic and "grates" the tomato.*

2 large slices toast, GF if necessary

1 garlic clove, halved

1 Roma tomato, halved

Salt

Nutritional yeast, optional

CRAZY MIXED-UP NUT BUTTER ON TOAST

MAKES: about 4 cups (about 755 g) nut butter
TIME: 10 minutes

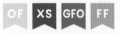

1 Pulse the nuts in a food processor until uniformly chopped. Transfer to a large bowl.

2 Stir in the seeds, then stir in the nut butter until thoroughly combined.

3 Spread some of the butter on the toast and serve. Transfer the rest to canning jars. Refrigerate to preserve the oils in the nuts and seeds, and use within 1 month.

NOTE: *Do not use a high-speed blender in step 1, or you'll end up with a super creamy nut butter! The fun is in the crunch.*

1⅔ cups (225 g) mixed nuts, preferably salted

½ cup (75 g) seeds: any combination of sunflower, pumpkin, sesame (toasted), chia, flax (ground), and hemp

One 16-ounce (454 g) jar creamy almond or peanut butter, preferably unsalted

Toast, GF if necessary, for serving

AVOCADO TOAST

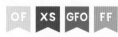

MAKES: 2 slices // **TIME:** 10 minutes

1 ripe avocado, halved,
    pitted, and sliced

2 large slices toast, GF if necessary

Salt, optional

Mash the avocado in a small bowl and spread onto the toast. Sprinkle with salt, if desired.

Variations: Avocado toast is wonderful when you first discover it, but it's easy to get bored with the plain variety. Here are a dozen new ways to top your toast and boost the nutrition and flavor of this quick breakfast.

1. Mild white or chickpea miso (spread on a thin layer before adding the avocado), plus a sprinkle of sesame seeds

2. Nutritional yeast and smoked paprika

3. Sliced tomato, black pepper, and red onion

4. Thinly sliced baked tofu (prepackaged or homemade)

5. Salsa (mashed with the avocado)

6. Sauerkraut or kimchi

7. A chiffonade (chopped into strips) of greens and a drizzle of balsamic

8. Cucumber slices and fresh dill

9. Chopped scallions and shredded carrots

10. Mashed chickpeas or white beans

11. Fresh herbs such as basil, mint, cilantro, or parsley, plus a squeeze of lemon or lime juice

12. Mashed roasted or black (fermented) garlic

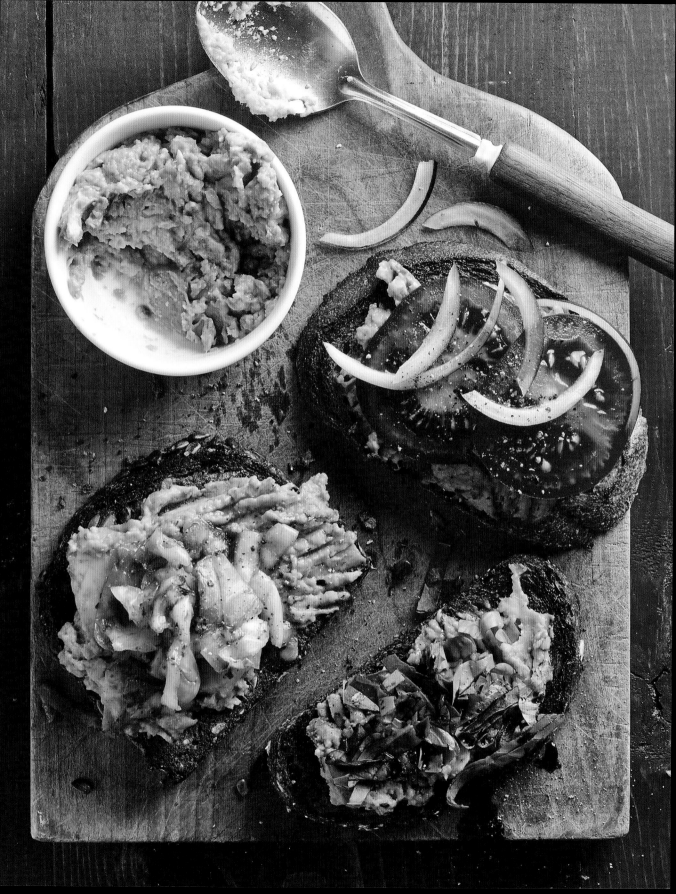

RISE & SHINE SALAD

MAKES: 1 to 2 salads // **TIME:** 15 minutes,
not including time to make Maple-Dijon Dressing,
Quick Pickled Onions, and Breakfast Hummus

Salad for breakfast? Yep. And why not? This hearty "salad" was created for those who just can't do something sweet first thing in the morning. You can really consider this to be a template for a salad that tastes like a savory breakfast. Use any greens or leftover roasted veggies you have. You can even swap in another dressing. Prep the ingredients ahead of time for breakfast in mere minutes.

1 bunch kale, stemmed and chopped into bite-size pieces

½ cup (120 ml) Maple-Dijon Dressing (page 154)

¼ cup (40 g) Quick Pickled Onions (page 240)

¼ cup (35 g) roasted sunflower or pumpkin seeds

1 large sweet potato, cubed and roasted

½ cup (115 g) Breakfast Hummus (page 56)

Place the kale in a medium bowl. Add the dressing and massage until the kale is dark green and shiny, about 5 minutes. Add the pickled onions, sunflower seeds, and sweet potato. Toss to combine and transfer to a bowl (or bowls). Top with the hummus and serve.

NOTE: *Boost the protein with a serving of Tempeh Breakfast Sausage (page 63).*

THE DAILY GRINDER

MAKES: 1 baguette, enough for 4 sandwiches // **TIME:** 15 minutes,
not including time to make Breakfast Hummus and Quick Pickled Onions

Sandwiches are quick breakfasts, and this one stays together on the go and stores well, too. (They're not too saucy and the ingredients are layered so there's "glue"—in the form of hummus—on the top and bottom.) You can make it the night before and reheat it in the toaster oven as is or wait until the morning to put the "wet" veggies on. It tastes particularly good after a long early morning workout.

1 Slice the baguette in half lengthwise, then slice each piece in half horizontally. Scoop out some of the insides, reserving them for another use (such as bread crumbs). (This makes more room for the filling.) Toast the bread lightly.

2 Spread the hummus inside both baguette halves; place the mixed vegetables, pickled onions, sprouts, and greens on the bottom baguette half. Add the avocado and plenty of hot sauce, if using. Top with the remaining baguette half.

3 Slice into sandwiches and serve or wrap tightly in foil until ready to eat.

1 sourdough or whole grain baguette

1 cup (225 g) Breakfast Hummus (page 56)

1 cup (110 g) mixed vegetables such as shredded carrots, cucumber slices, and/or bell pepper rings

½ cup (80 g) Quick Pickled Onions (page 240)

½ cup (15 g) alfalfa sprouts

4 cups (115 g) mixed baby greens

1 avocado, sliced, optional

Hot sauce, optional

SHIITAKE BAKIN'

MAKES: about 1 cup (about 85 g) // **TIME:** 35 minutes

Use this quick bacon stand-in on veggie burgers, atop mac and cheese, or in our BLAT Pita (page 71). You can also toss it with popcorn, sprinkle it on a baked potato, or use it to garnish a tofu scramble. Thinner slices will yield crispier bakin', so practice your knife skills with this recipe. If you're not using oil, the mushrooms will stay chewy rather than become crisp.

One 3.5-ounce (100 g) package shiitake mushrooms (stems discarded), sliced as thinly as possible (see Note)

1 tablespoon olive oil (OF: omit)

1 teaspoon maple syrup

1 teaspoon reduced-sodium, GF tamari

¼ teaspoon black pepper

¼ teaspoon garlic powder

¼ teaspoon smoked paprika

Tip: There are two schools of thought on cleaning mushrooms: rinse or wipe. The argument against rinsing is that the mushrooms will discolor and get slimy. On the other hand, wiping seems unsanitary to some. If they seem particularly dirty, it's fine to go ahead and give them a rinse in a colander. But if your mushrooms are fairly clean, you can simply wipe them with a lint-free towel or clean paintbrush to remove any debris.

1 Preheat the oven to 375°F (190°C). Line a baking sheet with parchment paper.

2 Combine the shiitakes, oil, maple syrup, tamari, pepper, garlic powder, and paprika in a medium bowl.

3 Spread the mushrooms in a single layer and bake for 30 minutes, tossing every 10 minutes, until the mushrooms start to crisp. Remove from the oven and allow to cool on the baking sheet before serving. (The mushrooms can be stored in an airtight container for up to 3 days.)

NOTE: Save clean shiitake stems for mushroom broth. They're too fibrous to eat, but they (and other mushroom stems) add flavor to broth.

TEMPEH BREAKFAST SAUSAGE

MAKES: 8 to 12 patties // **TIME:** 15 minutes to prep, 30 minutes to cook

This sausage takes center stage at brunch most weekends, usually next to a tofu scramble and roasted potatoes. Save any leftovers for your make-ahead breakfast burritos. We like Smiling Hara Black-Eyed Pea Tempeh, which also makes this recipe soy-free. Lightly steaming the tempeh reduces its bitterness.

1 Preheat the oven to 400°F (200°C). Line a baking sheet with parchment paper.

2 Place the tempeh in the bowl of a food processor. Add the maple syrup, flour, oil, miso, sage, rosemary, black pepper, and crushed red pepper and pulse to combine.

3 Transfer to a medium bowl and, using wet hands, form the mixture into 8 burger-size patties or 12 slider-size ones.

4 Place the patties on the prepared baking sheet and bake for 30 minutes (for burger-size patties) or 20 minutes (for slider-size patties), flipping halfway through. Serve. (The sausage can be refrigerated for up to 5 days.)

Variation: Turn this into sausage gravy by sautéing the sausage in a skillet, breaking it into chunks as it cooks. Once cooked, add ½ cup (120 ml) Miso Gravy (page 231) and ½ cup (120 ml) almond milk. Cook until thick and bubbly, about 5 minutes, and serve over roasted potatoes or Breakfast Tofu (page 65).

One 8-ounce (227 g) package tempeh, lightly steamed if desired, cubed

2 tablespoons maple syrup

2 tablespoons whole wheat flour

1 tablespoon olive oil (OF: 2 tablespoons broth)

1 tablespoon red miso

1 teaspoon dried sage

½ teaspoon dried rosemary

¼ teaspoon black pepper

⅛ teaspoon crushed red pepper

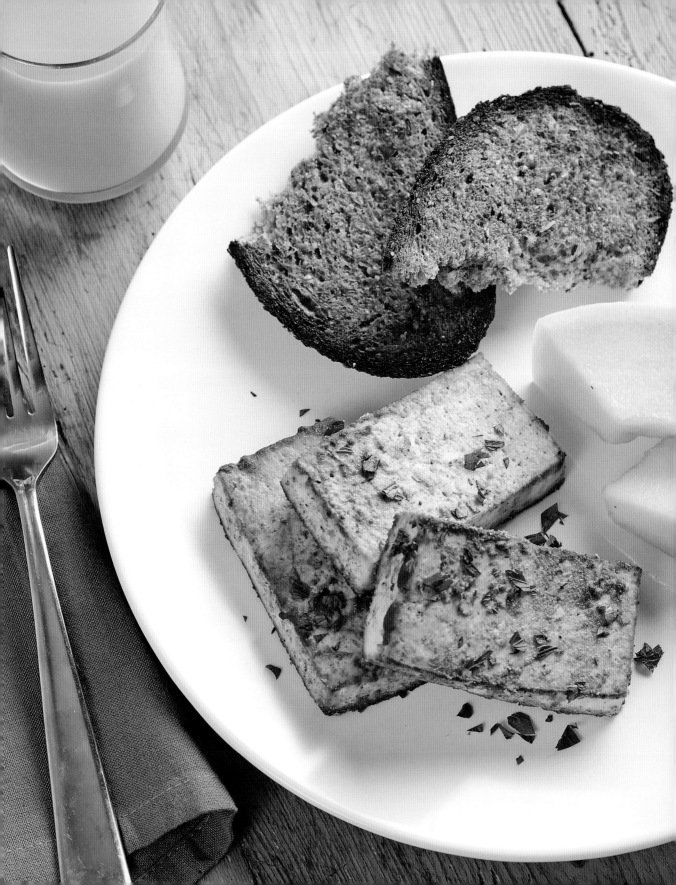

BREAKFAST TOFU

MAKES: 12 slices // **TIME:** 10 minutes to prep, 30 minutes to cook

This breakfast tofu is a mobile version of a tofu scramble, which—while delicious—doesn't travel well and requires stovetop supervision. Wrap a couple of slices of this tofu in a brown rice tortilla, or sandwich it between two slices of sprouted grain bread with loads of arugula, avocado, and even a few leftover cold roasted root veggies. If you make a big batch on the weekend, you can have your weekday breakfasts prepped and ready to go in three minutes flat. Although we prefer to serve this tofu at room temperature or cold from the fridge (it firms up as it cools), it can be eaten right away, too.

1 Preheat the oven to 400°F (200°C). Line a baking sheet with parchment paper.

2 Slice each package of tofu into six pieces. Pat dry. Drizzle evenly with the tamari.

3 Combine the nutritional yeast, cumin, garlic powder, turmeric, curry powder, and black pepper in a large rectangular food storage container with a tight-fitting lid. Place the sliced tofu in the container and shake gently until all slices are covered. (You might need to open the container and rotate the slices a bit.) Let sit while the oven preheats. (The marinated tofu can be refrigerated for up to 1 day.)

4 Place tofu on the baking sheet. Spread any extra seasoning mix on top. Bake for 30 minutes, flipping halfway through.

5 Serve at room temperature or cold from the fridge.

Two 16-ounce (454 g) packages sprouted or extra-firm tofu, drained

1 tablespoon reduced-sodium, GF tamari

¼ cup (15 g) nutritional yeast

1 teaspoon ground cumin

½ teaspoon garlic powder

½ teaspoon ground turmeric

½ teaspoon yellow curry powder

¼ teaspoon black pepper

ASSEMBLY-LINE BREAKFAST BURRITOS

When you're trying to jam a lot of things into your day, you learn to focus only on what you can control. And while you may not be able to change the fact that you need to get up early, breakfast is one thing over which you have total control. If you run around like crazy in the morning trying to get ready for a day of workouts, work, and errands, these make-ahead burritos are for you.

Spend an hour on the weekend prepping these burritos, and your weekday mornings will feel a little easier. Beyond breakfast, this big-batch meal saves the day whenever you need a quick bite.

TIPS:

1. Prep all your ingredients ahead of time and let them cool a bit. This will make burrito assembly easier.

2. Warm your tortillas or wraps to make them more pliable.

3. Keep the filling as dry as possible to avoid a soggy burrito.

4. If your burrito rolling technique isn't perfect, don't worry. As they cool, they will seal a bit better.

5. Burritos can be frozen for up to three months (though they likely won't last that long). Once each one is wrapped and allowed to cool, place in a freezer bag or an airtight container.

6. For best results, defrost in the fridge overnight, then microwave until warmed through, about 1 minute. You can also bake in a toaster oven at 350°F (180°C) until warmed through, 10 to 15 minutes.

EASY BEAN BURRITOS

MAKES: 12 burritos // **TIME:** 1 hour to prep, not including time to make Slow-Cooker Refried Beans

1 Drain any excess liquid from the sautéed vegetables. Mix the beans, sautéed vegetables, sweet potato, nutritional yeast, and salsa together in a bowl. Set aside.

2 Set up an assembly line on the counter with the tortillas, hummus, bean-vegetable mixture, and 12 squares of parchment paper or aluminum foil.

3 Working one at a time, warm the tortillas. (Microwave them for about 15 seconds each, or bake them at 350°F/180°C for 5 to 7 minutes wrapped in a damp, lint-free towel.)

4 Spread hummus on a warm tortilla, then top with heaping ½ cup (90 g) of the bean-vegetable mixture. Roll, starting by folding the bottom and top in, then the sides in. Wrap tightly in the parchment or foil. Repeat with the remaining tortillas and filling. Allow to cool, then refrigerate for up to 5 days or freeze for up to 2 months.

FF: *Use store-bought hummus and canned beans that have been drained and rinsed.*

Sautéed vegetables (choose one or more to yield 1 to 2 cups/150 to 300 g), such as:

- » 2 bell peppers, any color
- » 1 small onion
- » 1 bunch kale, leaves only
- » One 10-ounce (283 g) container cremini mushrooms

1½ cups (390 g) Slow-Cooker Refried Beans (page 174)

1 large sweet potato, cubed and roasted or steamed

½ cup (30 g) nutritional yeast

½ cup (120 g) salsa

12 (8-inch or 20 cm) whole-grain tortillas

1 cup (245 g) hummus or 1 cup (240 ml) Cashew Queso (page 237)

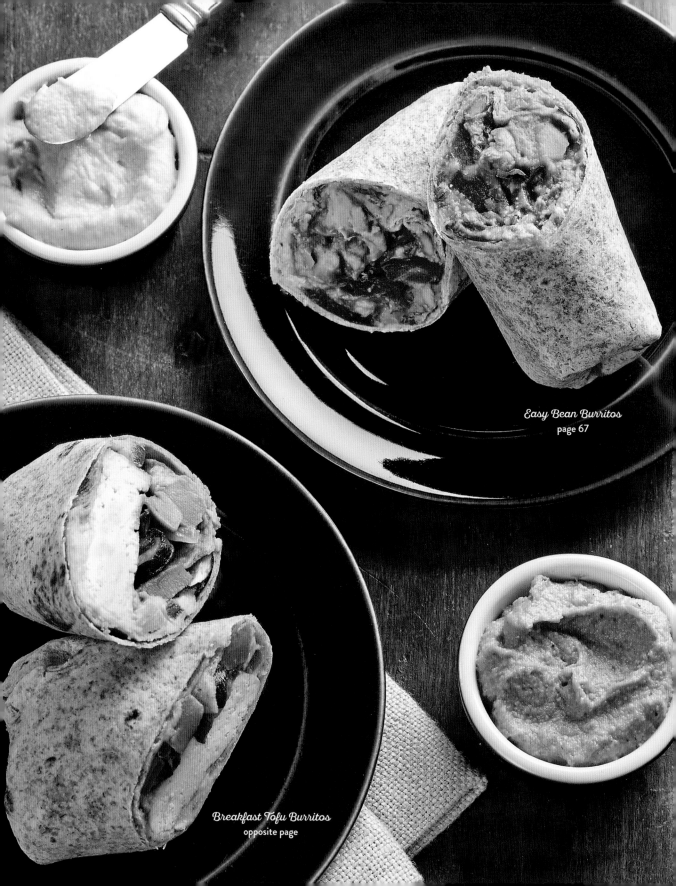

Easy Bean Burritos
page 67

Breakfast Tofu Burritos
opposite page

BREAKFAST TOFU BURRITOS

MAKES: 12 burritos // **TIME:** 1 hour to prep, not including time to make Breakfast Tofu

1 Drain any excess liquid from the sautéed vegetables. Mix the sautéed vegetables and sweet potatoes together in a bowl with the nutritional yeast.

2 Set up an assembly line on the counter with the tortillas, hummus, tofu, vegetables, and 12 squares of parchment paper or aluminum foil.

3 Working one at a time, warm the tortillas. (Microwave them for about 15 seconds each, or bake them at 350°F/180°C for 5 to 7 minutes wrapped in a damp, lint-free towel.)

4 Spread hummus on a warm tortilla, then top with 1 slice of tofu and ½ cup (90 g) veggie mixture. Roll, starting by folding the bottom and top in, then the sides. Wrap tightly in the parchment or foil. Repeat with the remaining tortillas and filling. Allow to cool, then refrigerate for up to 5 days or freeze for up to 2 months.

Sautéed vegetables (choose one or more to yield 1 to 2 cups/150 to 300 g), such as:

» 2 bell peppers, any color

» 1 small onion

» 1 bunch kale, leaves only

» One 10-ounce (283 g) package cremini mushrooms

1 large sweet potato, cubed and roasted or steamed

½ cup (30 g) nutritional yeast

12 (8-inch or 20 cm) whole-grain tortillas

1 cup (240 g) hummus or Cashew Queso (page 237)

12 slices Breakfast Tofu (page 65)

CHICKPEA QUICHE

MAKES: 2 quiches, each serving 4 to 6 // **TIME:** 10 minutes to prep, 45 minutes to bake

Chickpea flour (garbanzo bean or gram flour) is a favorite breakfast ingredient, as it makes a good substitute for eggs. You can whip up savory pancakes or flatbread with it, and we're quite partial to this quiche because you can make it ahead of time—and it travels well, too! Customize it as you would a frittata. If you're adding "wet" veggies such as onions, peppers, or mushrooms, sauté them first so you don't end up with soggy quiches.

2 cups (240 g) chickpea flour (garbanzo bean or gram flour)

¼ cup (15 g) nutritional yeast

1 teaspoon GF baking powder

½ teaspoon salt

¼ teaspoon ground turmeric

⅛ teaspoon black pepper

2 cups finely chopped greens, such as (30 g) kale, (70 g) collards, or (60 g) spinach

3 garlic cloves, minced

2 cups (480 ml) water

1 tablespoon olive oil, plus extra for greasing the plates (OF: omit)

1 Preheat the oven to 400°F (200°C). Coat two pie plates with olive oil (OF: use silicone cake pans).

2 Combine the flour, yeast, baking powder, salt, turmeric, and pepper in a large bowl. Stir in the greens and garlic, then whisk in the water and olive oil. The batter should be the consistency of pancake batter. (The batter can be refrigerated overnight. You might need to add up to ¼ cup/60 ml more water to thin it out the next morning.)

3 Pour in the batter and bake for 45 minutes, or until cooked through and a toothpick inserted in the middle comes out clean. Remove from the oven and let cool for 15 minutes. Slice into wedges and serve. (Leftovers can be stored, wrapped in parchment paper, for up to 3 days.)

Tip: You don't want this to be doughy in the middle. Doughy chickpea flour = uncooked legumes, which can cause GI distress.

HARISSA BAKED TOFU

SERVES: 2 to 4 // **TIME:** 20 minutes to prep, 30 minutes to bake

This tofu version of shakshuka, the traditional North African braised egg dish, is one of the few savory breakfasts that *isn't* so portable. However, this is a breakfast worth staying put for. The tofu soaks up the flavors of the spiced tomato sauce, which you'll want to sop up with toast, polenta, or a Rosemary–Black Pepper Scone (page 53).

1 Preheat the oven to 400°F (200°C).

2 Place a large, deep ovenproof skillet over medium heat. Add the oil and swirl to coat the pan, then add the onion. Cook, stirring often, until the onion starts to soften, about 5 minutes. Add the bell peppers and garlic and cook for 3 minutes longer. Add the harissa and turmeric and cook until fragrant, about 2 minutes.

3 Add the tomato paste and cook for 1 minute, stirring often, until it darkens. Stir in the tomatoes with their juice, the water, and salt, nestle the tofu in the sauce, and increase the heat to medium-high. Once the tomatoes start to bubble, remove from the heat, cover, and transfer to the oven.

4 Bake for 15 minutes, remove the lid, and continue to bake for 15 minutes more, until the tomato sauce is bubbly. Serve.

1 tablespoon olive oil (OF:
¼ cup/60 ml broth)

1 yellow onion, chopped fine

1 red or yellow bell pepper,
chopped fine

3 garlic cloves, minced

1 tablespoon Harissa (page 227)

¼ teaspoon ground turmeric

2 tablespoons tomato paste

One 28-ounce (794 g) can diced
tomatoes with juice

1 cup (240 ml) water

¼ teaspoon salt

Two 16-ounce (454 g) packages
sprouted or extra-firm tofu,
drained and sliced into 12 pieces

Chapter 4

DINNERS & HEARTY MEALS TO FUEL & AID RECOVERY

After working all day and then working out, you want something filling and rewarding that doesn't take all night to prepare. Hearty dinners like Beet Bourguignon (Beet & Lentil Stew—page 125), Buddha Bowls (page 89), and Roasted Red Pepper Mac & Cheese (page 117) help you repair and recover—while still satisfying the rest of the family—so you can get out there the next day to do it all again.

It's repeated so often it's almost a cliché, but it's on target so we'll say it again: Though many people look at a plant-based diet as a restrictive one—one that simply eliminates foods—anyone who has actually adopted it knows that the opposite is true. When you can no longer rely on the old meat-and-potato standbys, suddenly you're forced to branch out into new and unexplored ways of eating—and the result is dozens of (or maybe even a hundred) new foods in your diet.

You start planning your meals around what's in season at the farmers market. You spend most of your shopping time in the produce section, seeking out unknown, exotic fruits and vegetables you once ignored. Maybe you even discover your local Asian or Indian market and have a field day the first time you go.

And because places like Outback and Red Lobster no longer hold much appeal for you, you branch out and discover the Korean restaurant that you've never bothered to try or the simply amazing Ethiopian place you didn't even realize was nearby.

This experience is what we tried to capture in the list of recipes that make up this cookbook, and in particular this section of main dishes. You'll notice a lot of international influences, though we've given most recipes names that will sound more familiar. Without the grilled meat, bulgogi sauce evolved into Korean Tahini BBQ Sauce (page 230), and the Ethiopian stew *shiro wot* became Chickpea "Polenta" Stew (page 91). We've taken inspiration from dishes around the globe, streamlining them to fit into our schedules, our pantry lists, and our personal taste.

Since plant-based eating is a lifestyle for us, we've discovered naturally meat-free and "veganized" fare the world over during our respective travels. We love the experience of being introduced to new foods, and it is these experiences (and recipe inspiration) that we bring home from trips near and far.

Many international cuisines simply lend themselves more easily to plant-based eating than typical American fare does. In Japan, fish is a staple, and in Korea, pork is incredibly popular, but vegetables and grains (albeit typically white rice) still make up more than half of most meals. Spanish-style tapas, Turkish breakfast feasts, and Guatemalan rice-and-bean platters all use meat sparingly, making it an easy ingredient to omit when cooking such foods at home.

And, since food is about more than just fueling our bodies—it's history, community, and, in many cases, an act of love—recasting our favorite childhood meals and family specialties as plant-based dishes is a way to keep traditions alive. We've included plenty of those familiar, comforting recipes, too.

HEARTY VEGGIE HOAGIES

MAKES: 1 baguette, enough for 4 sandwiches // **TIME:** 15 minutes

This is a plant-based spin on a classic sandwich from southern France, *pan bagnat*. We ditched the traditional tuna but kept all the other flavors. If desired, spread a thin layer of hummus inside your baguette. This sandwich gets tastier the longer it marinates, so pack it in your jersey pocket or backpack and dig in midday.

One 12-ounce (340 g) sourdough or whole grain baguette

2 tomatoes, sliced

1 cucumber, sliced, salted, and drained

1 cup (260 g) canned or frozen and thawed artichoke hearts, roughly chopped

1 red bell pepper, sliced into rings

¼ small red onion, thinly sliced

⅓ cup (60 g) Kalamata olives, pitted and chopped

Salt and black pepper

2 tablespoons pesto (such as the one on page 233)

Balsamic vinegar

1 Slice the baguette in half horizontally (into two shorter segments), then slice off the top third from each half. Scoop out some of the insides of the bottom portion, reserving them for another use (such as bread crumbs).

2 Toast lightly.

3 Meanwhile, combine the tomatoes, cucumber, artichokes, bell pepper, onion, and olives in a medium bowl and season with salt and pepper to taste.

4 Spread the vegetables inside the bottom section of the baguette (being mindful not to add too much liquid).

5 Spread the pesto on the cut side of the baguette top. Drizzle the contents of the bottom with a bit of balsamic, then place the baguette top onto the vegetables.

6 Wrap tightly in parchment paper, then aluminum foil. For best flavor, let sit for at least 1 hour or up to 12 hours. Slice and serve.

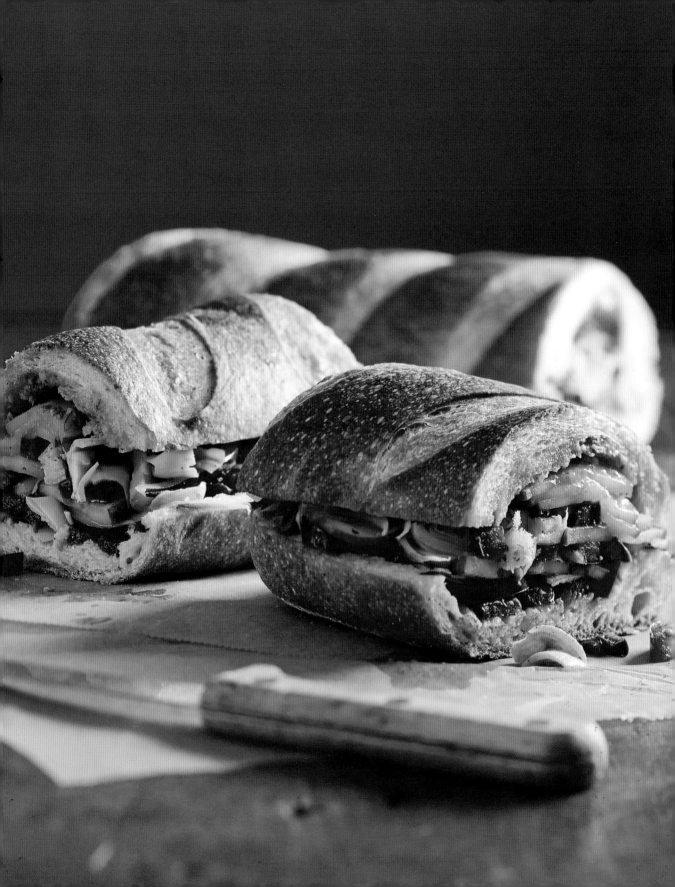

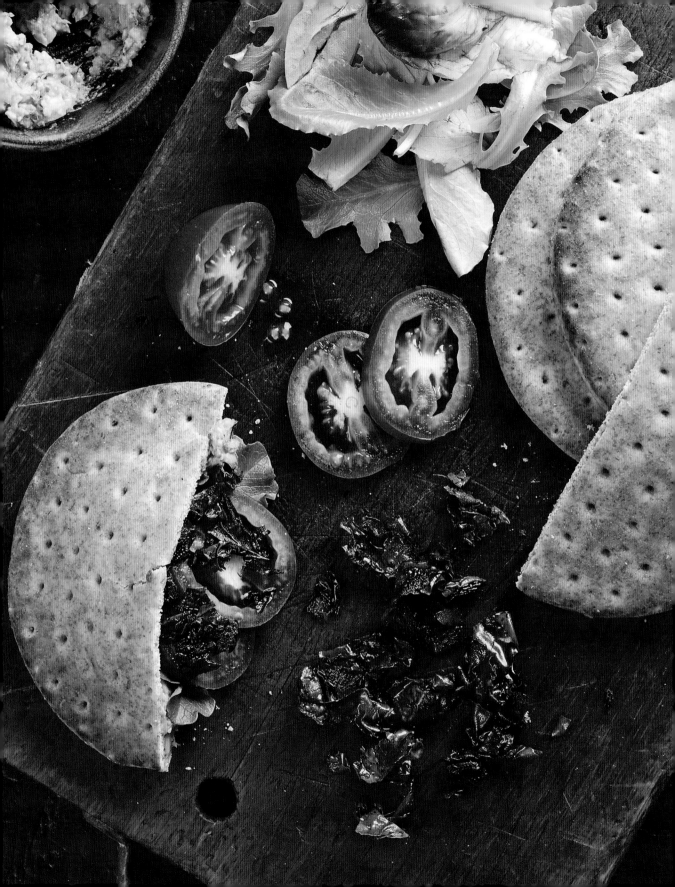

BLAT (BACON, LETTUCE, AVOCADO & TOMATO) PITAS

MAKES: 4 sandwiches // **TIME:** 20 minutes

There's a joke that vegans can make bacon out of anything, and we do—anything from mushrooms to coconut and even seaweed. Dulse is reddish-brown seaweed that grows in the northern Atlantic and Pacific. Like all sea veggies, it's a good source of vitamins and minerals, and it's high in protein by weight. When toasted, it takes on the texture of bacon. Here, we crumble it and stuff into a pita for a plant-based spin on the BLT! If you're not a fan of seaweed, you can substitute Shiitake Bakin' (page 62).

1 Place a large cast-iron skillet over medium heat. Once it's warm, add the coconut oil, then the dulse and liquid smoke. Toss to combine. Cook, stirring often, until the dulse is crispy, about 5 minutes. Remove from the heat and season with pepper to taste.

2 Mash the avocado with the cilantro, scallions, and lime juice. Season with salt and pepper to taste.

3 Slice the pitas in half and toast lightly. Gently open them, and divide the avocado mixture evenly into all 8 halves. Divide the greens, tomatoes, and dulse evenly among the pitas and serve.

NOTE: *Add a sprinkle of smoked paprika for an even smokier bacon taste. The crispy dulse itself is really good on popcorn with nutritional yeast, salt, and pepper.*

2 teaspoons coconut oil (OF: omit)

½ cup (10 g) dulse, picked through and separated, or 1 batch Shiitake Bakin' (page 62)

Few drops liquid smoke

Salt and black pepper

2 avocados, sliced

¼ cup (5 g) chopped cilantro

2 scallions (white and light green parts), sliced

2 tablespoons lime juice

Four 8-inch (20 cm) whole wheat pitas

4 cups (115 g) greens (mixed baby greens or chopped romaine)

4 plum tomatoes, sliced

LOADED SPAGHETTI SQUASH

MAKES: 2 stuffed halves // **TIME:** 55 minutes

Squash is like nature's bowl; it's just begging to be stuffed. Here, we loaded up on everything we'd normally put on pasta for a fun, quick dinner. This is one that's regularly added to the menu in winter, with the squash prepped on a batch-cooking day. Bake your squash ahead of time so dinner can be quick.

1 large spaghetti squash

Salt and black pepper

Dried herbs, such as oregano, basil, or fennel

2 roasted red peppers, chopped

2 cups (55 g) baby spinach, chopped

1 cup (165 g) cooked chickpeas

½ cup (130 g) canned or frozen and thawed artichoke hearts, roughly chopped

¼ cup (45 g) pitted Kalamata olives, chopped

¼ cup (15 g) sun-dried tomatoes (not packed in oil), chopped

1 cup (250 g) jarred pasta sauce or Weeknight Marinara (page 81)

Chopped basil

Cashew Cream (page 236), optional

❶ Preheat the oven to 400°F (200°C). Line a baking sheet with parchment paper.

❷ Slice the squash in half, scoop out the seeds, then sprinkle the inside liberally with salt, pepper, and herbs of your choice. Place cut side down on the baking sheet. Bake about 30 minutes, or until the squash is fork-tender and cooked through. At this point, you can let the squash cool and refrigerate until ready to eat.

❸ While the squash is baking or when you're ready to eat, combine the red peppers, greens, chickpeas, artichoke hearts, olives, and sun-dried tomatoes in a medium bowl.

❹ Spread half the marinara inside the squash halves, then divide the vegetables between the squash halves.

❺ Top with the remaining marinara and bake for 15 minutes, until the squash is heated through and the sauce is bubbly. Sprinkle with the basil and serve with the cashew cream, if using.

NOTE: *Some cooking methods call for poaching squash in water, but this can yield mushy, bland, watery squash. This version allows for some color on the cut side, and by baking it cut side down, you seal in moisture.*

FF: *Stop by the grocery store olive bar for small amounts of roasted peppers, sun-dried tomatoes, and, of course, olives.*

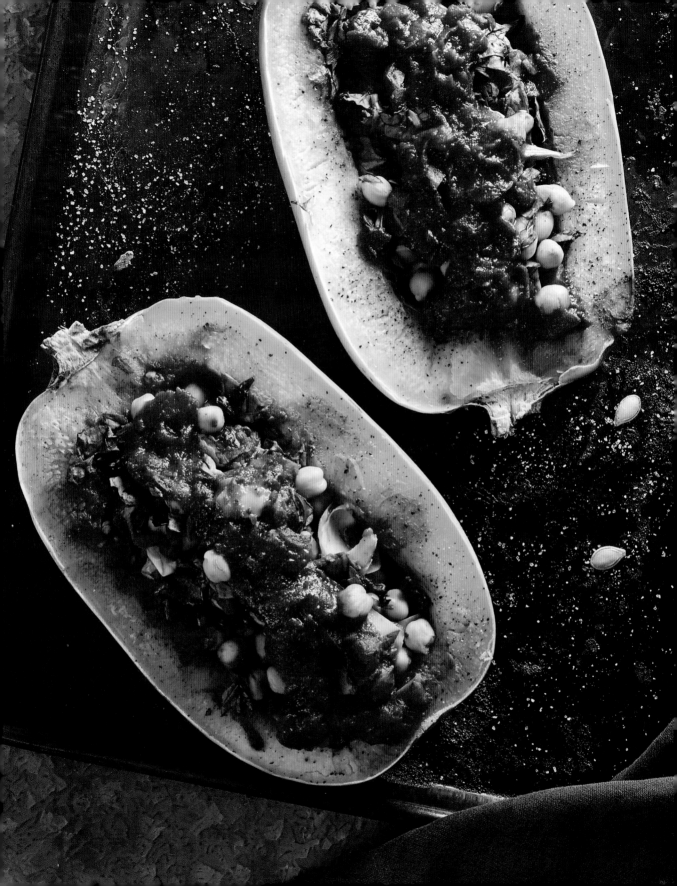

ONE-POT PASTA

SERVES: 2 to 4 // **TIME:** 25 minutes

One-pot pastas are all the rage, and now that we've made one, we can see why! You only dirty one pot, and the sauce is thick and creamy; it's a quick meal disguised as comfort food. You may doubt the magic of the single pot the first time, but as long as you stir, stir, stir, you'll be a convert with the first bite. While you can use long pasta like spaghetti, it's a bit trickier to keep from sticking. If you only have a long, stringy pasta at home, break it into 2-inch (5 cm) pieces first.

16 ounces (454 g) small whole wheat pasta, such as penne, farfalle, or macaroni, or GF if necessary

5 cups (1.2 L) water

One 15-ounce (425 g) can cannellini beans, drained and rinsed

One 14.5-ounce (411 g) can diced (with juice) or crushed tomatoes

1 yellow onion, chopped

1 red or yellow bell pepper, chopped

2 tablespoons tomato paste

1 tablespoon Italian Spices (page 224)

1 tablespoon olive oil (OF: ¼ cup/60 ml broth)

3 garlic cloves, minced

¼ teaspoon crushed red pepper, optional

1 bunch kale, stemmed and chopped

1 cup (42 g) sliced basil (see Note)

½ cup (90 g) pitted Kalamata olives, chopped

1 Add the pasta, water, beans, tomatoes (with juice if using diced), onion, bell pepper, tomato paste, Italian spices, oil, garlic, and crushed red pepper, if using, to a large stockpot or deep skillet with a lid. Bring to a boil over high heat, stirring often.

2 Reduce the heat to medium-high, add the kale, and cook, continuing to stir often, until the pasta is al dente, about 10 minutes. (Seriously: Do *not* forget to stir or the pasta will clump and thicken. If you neglect your duties and this does happen, add ¼ cup/60 ml water or broth to loosen.)

3 Remove from the heat and let sit for 5 minutes (now you can stop stirring). Garnish with the basil and olives and serve.

NOTE: *To slice the basil, stack the leaves, roll them into a cigarlike shape, and slice into ribbons.*

Tip: Save time by boiling water in an electric kettle while you do your prep work. Add to the pot and proceed as directed.

PASTA MARINARA WITH SPICY ITALIAN BEAN BALLS

SERVES: 2 to 4 / Makes about 3 cups (720 g) marinara // **TIME:** 20 minutes to prep, 30 minutes to bake

There are so many interesting vegan meat swaps on the market these days, but most are made with ingredients we don't consider to be whole foods. These are a cleaner version of meatballs that taste like pepperoni, at least from what we remember. They're soy-free and can easily be made gluten-free by using gluten-free bread crumbs, and the dish can be made gluten-free by using gluten-free pasta or omitting pasta altogether.

For days when you don't want the jarred stuff but also don't want to spend all day simmering sauce, just make this Weeknight Marinara, adding bean balls if you've prepped them ahead of time. It works with fresh or canned tomatoes, and it's ready in just about the time it takes to boil pasta and open a can of beans. If your tomatoes are unsalted, you can add ¼ teaspoon salt before serving.

1 **To make the bean balls,** preheat the oven to 350°F (180°C). Line a baking sheet with parchment paper (see Note).

2 Heat a medium skillet over medium heat, then add the olive oil. Add the onion and cook, stirring often, until it begins to soften, about 5 minutes.

2 Add the oregano, fennel seeds, garlic powder, and crushed red pepper. Cook until fragrant, about 1 minute longer. Remove from the heat and transfer to a food processor along with the beans.

3 Pulse to combine and season with salt and pepper to taste; add the bread crumbs. Pulse until just combined.

4 Using a 2-ounce (3 to 4 tablespoon) cookie scoop, form balls (it may be necessary to wet hands to prevent sticking). Bake for 15 minutes, flip, and bake 15 minutes longer, or until golden brown.

Recipe and ingredients continue . . .

SPICY ITALIAN BEAN BALLS

1 tablespoon olive oil (OF: ¼ cup/60 ml broth)

½ yellow onion, minced

2 teaspoons dried oregano

1 teaspoon fennel seeds

1 teaspoon garlic powder

½ teaspoon crushed red pepper

One 15-ounce (425 g) can white beans (cannellini or navy), drained and rinsed

Salt and black pepper

½ cup (30 g) whole-grain bread crumbs (GF if necessary)

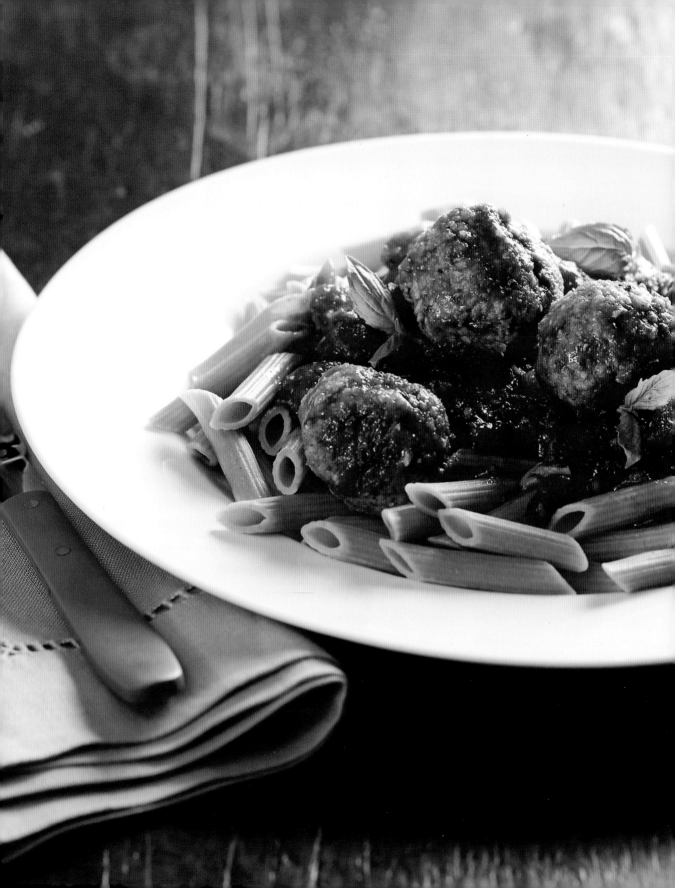

5 **Meanwhile, make the marinara:** Place a medium saucepan over medium-high heat. Add the oil to the hot pan. Once it's warm, add the basil and garlic and cook for 2 minutes, stirring occasionally. Stir in the tomatoes with their juice, bring just to a boil, then reduce heat to low, cover, and cook for 15 minutes. Season with salt, if desired.

6 Cook the pasta according to package instructions. Serve topped with the bean balls and marinara sauce.

NOTE: *To eliminate oil when baking, we use unbleached parchment paper on our baking sheets. If you prefer, you can grease your baking sheets or use a silicone liner. Do not substitute wax paper, which will burn (and make your food taste like crayons).*

Variation: For a Sardinian-style sauce, add 1 teaspoon fennel seeds with the garlic.

WEEKNIGHT MARINARA

1 tablespoon olive oil (OF: 2 tablespoons mushroom stock)

Handful basil leaves

3 garlic cloves, minced

One 28-ounce (794 g) can whole tomatoes with juice reserved, tomatoes pureed or chopped

Salt (optional)

Pasta, GF if necessary, as desired

LENTIL-MUSHROOM NO-MEAT PASTA (BOLOGNESE)

SERVES: 2 to 4 / Makes about 6 cups (1.4 kg) sauce // **TIME:** 1 hour

Lots of people have fond childhood associations with spaghetti and meat sauce, and there's no reason you can't get that same comfort from a plant-based version! The combination of lentils and mushrooms (vegan-*ese*, if you will) contributes plenty of flavor and a hearty texture to this simple pasta sauce. Serve over whole-grain pasta or polenta. It freezes well and can easily be multiplied to serve a crowd. Leftovers can be served atop simple oats in the morning, too.

2 tablespoons olive oil (OF:
 ¼ cup/60 ml mushroom stock)

1 large yellow onion, finely diced

2 portobello mushrooms or one
 10-ounce (283 g) package
 cremini mushrooms, trimmed
 and chopped fine

2 tablespoons tomato paste

3 garlic cloves, chopped

1 teaspoon oregano

2½ cups (600 ml) water

1 cup (200 g) brown lentils

One 28-ounce (794 g) can pureed
 or diced tomatoes with basil
 (with juice if diced)

1 tablespoon balsamic vinegar

Pasta

Salt and black pepper

Chopped basil

1 Place a large stockpot over medium heat. Add the oil. Once the oil is hot (or the broth starts to simmer), add the onion and mushrooms. Cover and cook until both are soft, about 5 minutes. Add the tomato paste, garlic, and oregano and cook 2 minutes, stirring constantly.

2 Stir in the water and lentils. Bring to a boil, then reduce the heat to medium-low and cook for 5 minutes, covered. Add the tomatoes (and juice if using diced) and vinegar. Replace the lid, reduce the heat to low and cook until the lentils are tender, about 30 minutes.

3 Cook the pasta according to the package instructions.

4 Remove the sauce from the heat and season with salt and pepper to taste. Garnish with the basil and serve atop the pasta.

FF: *Use precooked lentils, which are available in cans or in sealed packages in the refrigerated vegetable cooler. Omit the water in the recipe if you take this route, and cook the sauce over medium-low for 20 minutes, stirring in the lentils at the end just to heat them.*

NOTE: *Always examine your legumes—lentils, beans, and their brethren—before using them in a recipe. If they are cracked, wrinkly, or otherwise weird-looking, they may take longer to cook. In some cases, they may not soften at all. (Skip them and open a can of beans for dinner instead!)*

Variation: Substitute ½ cup (50 g) finely chopped walnuts for the mushrooms.

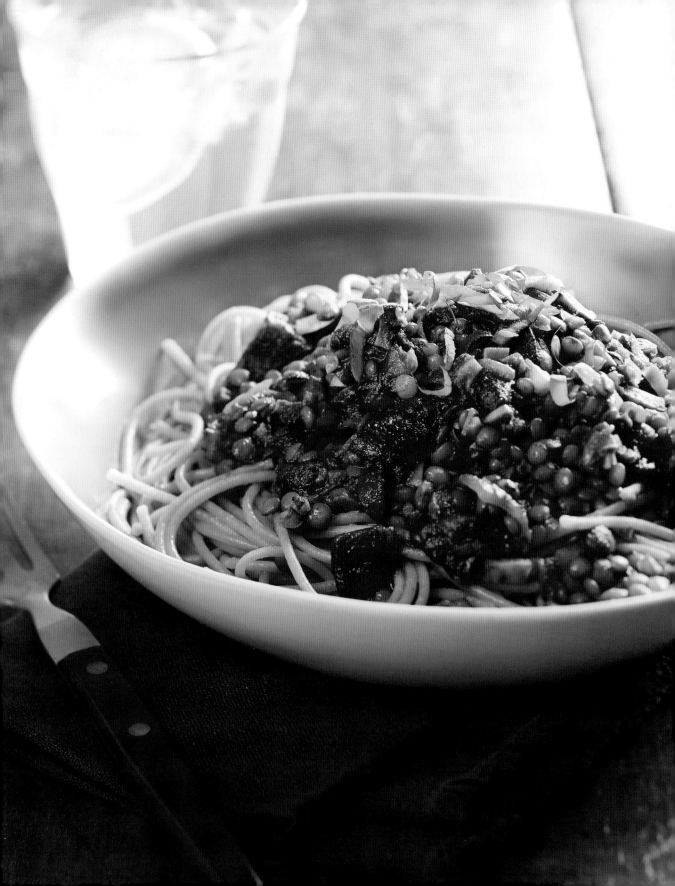

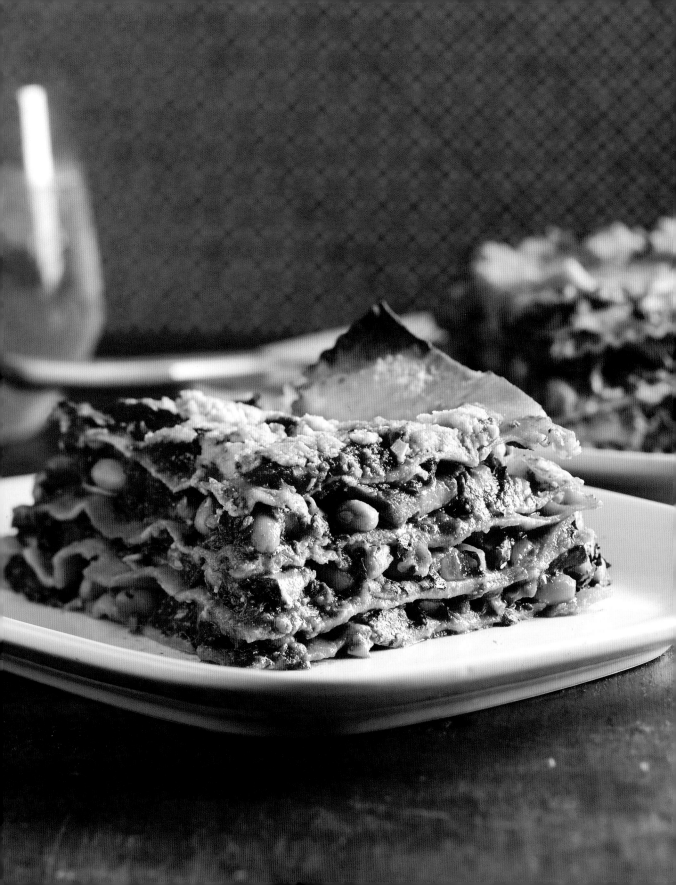

SIMPLIFIED SPINACH-MUSHROOM LASAGNA

MAKES: one 9 x 13-inch (23 x 33 cm) lasagna // **TIME:** 30 minutes to prep, 1 hour to bake, not including time to make Cashew Cream

Lasagna is definitely not a quick meal, but it's worth the effort and feeds a crowd. This version uses no vegan analogs or processed foods; instead, it's full of whole food versions of the traditional ingredients. Be sure to use a good jarred sauce (or our Weeknight Marinara).

1 Preheat the oven to 400°F (200°C). Place a large skillet over medium heat. Add the oil, then the onion and garlic. Sauté, stirring often, until the onions are soft and starting to color, about 10 minutes. (OF: Add more broth as needed.) Transfer half of the onion mixture to a medium bowl and set aside.

2 Add the mushrooms, oregano, fennel seeds, and ¼ teaspoon salt to the remaining onion mixture in the skillet. (OF: Add another splash of broth.) Cook, stirring often, until the mushrooms are dark and have released their liquid, about 10 minutes. Remove from the heat.

3 While the mushrooms cook, add the beans, spinach, nutritional yeast, and remaining ¼ teaspoon salt to the bowl with the onion mixture. Combine thoroughly.

4 Spread 1 cup (240 g) of the sauce in the bottom of a 9 x 13-inch (23 x 33 cm) pan. Top with a layer of noodles, one third of the spinach-bean mixture, one third of the mushroom mixture and 1 cup (240 g) sauce. (When you run out of sauce in each jar, add ½ cup/120 ml water, swirl it around, and set aside.) Repeat two more times, then top with a final layer of noodles and sauce. Add the water from the sauce jars, if using, around the edges, then top with the cashew cream.

5 Cover with parchment paper and an inverted baking sheet and bake for 40 minutes. Uncover and bake for another 10 minutes. Allow to cool for 20 minutes before slicing. Garnish with basil and the pesto, if using, and serve.

1 tablespoon olive oil (OF: ¼ cup/60 ml broth)

1 yellow onion, diced

2 garlic cloves, minced

Two 10-ounce (283 g) packages cremini mushrooms, trimmed and chopped

½ teaspoon dried oregano

½ teaspoon fennel seeds

½ teaspoon salt

3 cups (540 g) cooked white beans, or two 15-ounce (425 g) cans white beans, drained and rinsed

One 16-ounce (454 g) bag frozen spinach, thawed and squeezed dry in a lint-free towel

½ cup (30 g) nutritional yeast

One 9-ounce (255 g) box whole wheat no-boil lasagna noodles

Two 24-ounce (680 g) jars marinara sauce or 2 batches Weeknight Marinara (page 81)

1 batch Cashew Cream (page 236)

Chopped basil

Vegan Basil Pesto (page 233), optional

> **Tip:** Use a Microplane to grate a Brazil nut on top of pasta to yield mounds of fluffy, Parmesan-like ribbons.

BLUEPRINT: LIFESAVING BOWL

MAKES: 1 bowl, but easily scaled up // **TIME:** 10 minutes, not including time to cook quinoa

A cross between a salad and A Grain, a Green & a Bean (page 98), some nights these bowls are the only thing that stands between us and takeout. There's no recipe, just a formula—and a prayer of gratitude for their existence when you're starving and lacking the motivation to cook. If desired, crumble toasted dulse on top for more flavor.

1 cup (185 g) cooked quinoa or any GF whole grain

1 cup (110 g) shredded or chopped raw vegetables such as carrots, onions, bell peppers, and/or cucumbers

½ avocado, sliced, or ¼ cup (60 g) GF hummus or salsa

¼ cup (60 g) prepared sauerkraut or kimchi

2 tablespoons nutritional yeast

1 tablespoon lime juice or vinegar

Sesame or hemp seeds

Layer all the ingredients in a bowl and dig in.

BUDDHA BOWL

MAKES: 1 bowl, but easily scaled up for more Buddhas! // **TIME:** 15 minutes, not including time to cook quinoa or make Korean Tahini BBQ Sauce

In Asheville, North Carolina, we have several amazing vegan and vegetarian restaurants, but there's only one Rosetta's Kitchen. Rosetta's is an institution, having served up comfort food and hearty bowls brimming with local, organic vegetables since 2002. Rosetta's Buddha Bowl is fresh yet filling, and this is our attempt at re-creating it. If you're ever in Asheville, do yourself a favor and try the original, but in the meantime, this bowl of plenty will satisfy your belly and soul.

Warm the grains, tofu, and sauce and transfer to a bowl. Top with the remaining ingredients. Dig in!

1 cup (185 to 195 g) cooked quinoa or brown rice

4 ounces (115 g) tofu or tempeh— any variety (preferably baked after being marinated in the B-Savory Sauce & Marinade on page 232)

¼ cup (60 ml) Korean Tahini BBQ Sauce (page 230)

2 cups (60 g) mixed baby greens

½ cup (55 g) shredded carrots or beets

½ cup (105 g) mung bean sprouts

½ cup (115 g) sauerkraut or kimchi

½ avocado, sliced

Sesame or hemp seeds

JERK KIDNEY BEANS

SERVES: 2 to 4 // **TIME:** 15 minutes, not including time to cook rice

Confession: This started out as a semi-homemade meal, using half a jar of leftover tomato basil sauce and a can of red kidney beans. Turns out, adding jerk seasoning unites these two disparate ingredients so well that this is now a favorite quick weeknight meal served over rice or pasta with peas or steamed greens. If you like your food spicy, add another tablespoon or two of the Jerk Spices.

1 tablespoon coconut oil
(OF: ¼ cup/60 ml broth)

1 large yellow onion, diced

2 tablespoons Jerk Spices
(page 225)

One 14.5-ounce (411 g) can diced
tomatoes with juice

One 15-ounce (425 g) can red
kidney beans, drained and rinsed

Half a 24-ounce (680 g)
jar marinara sauce or one
14.5-ounce (411 g) can
tomato sauce

Salt and black pepper

Cooked brown rice
(½ cup/100 g per serving)

1 Place a medium saucepan over medium-high heat. Add the coconut oil. Once it melts, add the onion. Cook for 5 minutes, then stir in the jerk spices. Cook for 1 minute, then add the diced tomatoes with their juice, the beans, and marinara sauce. Bring to a simmer, cover, and cook for 10 minutes.

2 Season with salt and pepper to taste, and serve over the rice.

RED ALERT: *Red kidney beans can't be slow cooked. They contain a group of proteins (lectins) that is toxic unless cooked at a high temperature—and slow cooking isn't sufficient. Canned beans are safe, as they've been fully cooked at a proper temperature.*

CHICKPEA "POLENTA" STEW

SERVES: 2 to 4 // **TIME:** 40 minutes

This stew was inspired by our affinity for chickpea flour and the Ethiopian dish *shiro wot*. It yields a polenta-like stew that can be eaten as is (even for breakfast) or atop steamed veggies. Pair with pita wedges or rice for a more substantial meal.

Harissa (page 227) is used in the base recipe, but this dish works with almost every other seasoning blend listed in the beginning of the Flavor Boosts chapter (see pages 221–247).

1 Place a medium stockpot over medium heat. Add oil and the spice blend and cook until fragrant, about 1 minute. Add the onion and cook until beginning to soften, about 3 minutes.

2 Add the water and flour, then the tomatoes with their juice. Stir to combine, cover, and cook for 30 minutes, stirring every 10 minutes.

3 Remove from the heat and let sit for 10 minutes before serving.

1 tablespoon oil (OF: ¼ cup/60 ml broth)

2 tablespoons spice blend, such as Harissa (page 227)

1 yellow onion, chopped

2 cups (480 ml) water

1 cup (120 g) chickpea flour (garbanzo bean flour), soaked in water overnight

One 28-ounce (794 g) can diced tomatoes with juice

BLUEPRINT: BETTER THAN TAKEOUT CURRY

SERVES: 4 to 6 // **TIME:** 15 minutes to prep, 25 minutes to cook

This is finally it, an easy curry that's better than takeout! The secret? Sugar and salt. (Don't worry, it's only a bit of each.) Without them, the heat of the spices overwhelms the dish; the sugar and salt help round out the flavor. The fat from the coconut milk contributes creaminess and richness, providing a perfect foil to the spicy elements.

This curry is a formula. Throw in any vegetable that's in your crisper—the more, the merrier. You'll simply add the hard vegetables along with the potatoes and the softer ones later. If you don't have red lentils on hand, feel free use any cooked or canned bean. Eat this curry as is (it's a well-balanced meal) or with rice or naan.

1 tablespoon coconut oil
(OF: ¼ cup/60 ml broth)

1 red or yellow bell pepper, chopped

1 yellow onion, chopped

3 garlic cloves, minced

2 teaspoons Garam Masala
(page 223 or store-bought)

2 tablespoons yellow curry powder

2 tablespoons tomato paste

2 sweet potatoes, chopped

2 waxy potatoes, such as Yukon
Gold, chopped

2 carrots, chopped

1½ cups (310 g) red lentils, rinsed
and drained

4 cups (960 ml) water

1 small head cauliflower, broken
into florets

¼ cup (60 ml) light or full-fat
coconut milk

1 tablespoon dark brown sugar

1 tablespoon arrowroot powder

1 tablespoon lime juice

1 tablespoon red miso

Chopped basil or cilantro

1 Melt the coconut oil in a large stockpot over medium heat. Add the bell pepper, onion, and garlic and cook, stirring occasionally, until the vegetables are soft, about 3 minutes. Add the garam masala and curry powder, stir to combine, and cook until fragrant, about 1 minute.

2 Stir in the tomato paste. Cook, stirring often, until the tomato paste is fragrant and starting to darken, about 1 minute.

3 Add the sweet potatoes, waxy potatoes, carrots, and lentils. Stir to combine, then add the water and increase the heat to high. Bring just to a boil, then lower the heat to medium and stir in the cauliflower, coconut milk, and sugar.

4 Cover and cook until the vegetables are fork-tender, about 12 minutes. Remove from the heat.

5 In a small bowl, combine the arrowroot powder, lime juice, and miso, along with about ¼ cup (60 ml) liquid from the pot. Stir the mixture into the stew. Let cool until the sauce thickens, about 10 minutes. Sprinkle with basil and serve.

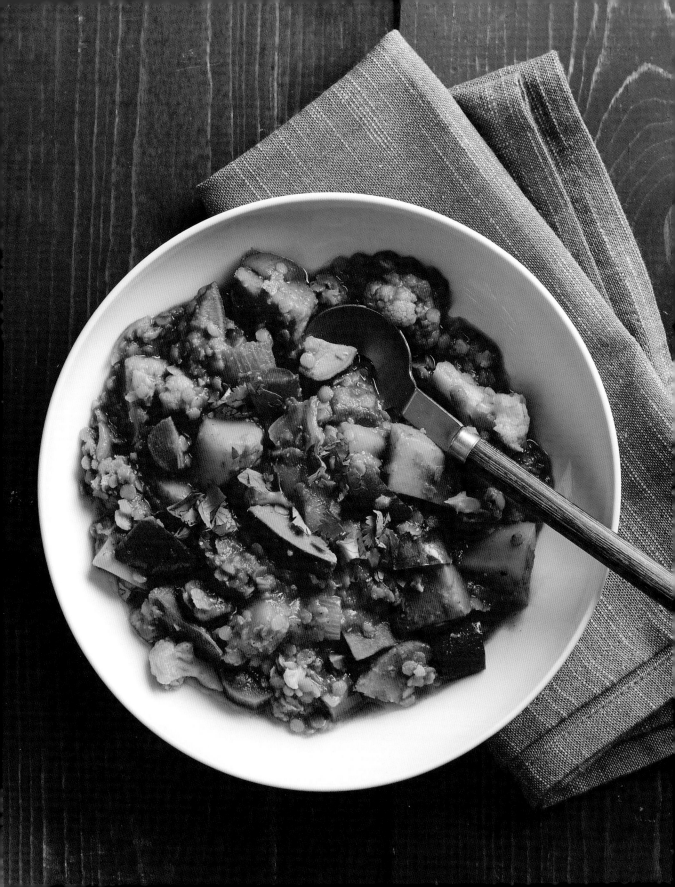

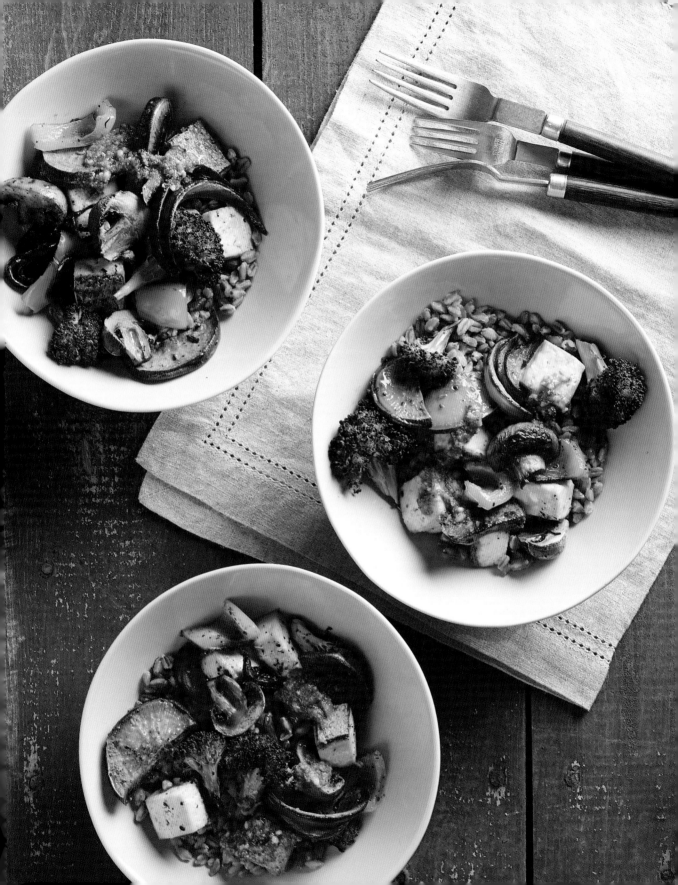

OFO GF

BLUEPRINT: SHEET-PAN MEALS (ROASTED VEGGIES WITH TOFU)

SERVES: 2 to 4 // **TIME:** 10 minutes to prep, 30 minutes to bake

There's something you don't realize about Asheville unless you've lived here a while: It's a temperate rainforest. It often rains suddenly (and hard!) in the afternoons and early evening throughout the summer—which means firing up the grill for dinner can be a gamble. This sheet-pan meal has become a stand-in for grilled summer dinners. While it doesn't lend the smoky char that the grill does (it turns out that's not so great for our health anyway), it does leave you with more time in the evening to squeeze in a workout.

Pair this simple dish with any sauce that complements your spice blend. See Chapter 5 (page 129) and Chapter 8 (page 221) for more ideas. We particularly like Miso Gravy (page 231), Classic French Vinaigrette (page 153), or Vegan Basil Pesto (page 233). This works equally well with tempeh.

1 Preheat the oven to 400°F (200°C). Line two baking sheets with parchment paper.

2 Chop the vegetables into equal-size pieces. Cube the tofu.

3 Divide the vegetables and tofu between the prepared baking sheets. Drizzle with the oil, and sprinkle the spices evenly over the baking sheets. Toss to thoroughly coat, and season with salt and pepper.

4 Bake, uncovered, until the vegetables are cooked through and starting to brown, about 30 minutes. (Rotate the baking sheets halfway through if necessary for even cooking.) Serve.

Tip: To prevent oil-free roasted vegetables from drying out, place a second piece of parchment or a silicone mat on top, along with another baking sheet. This will help seal in moisture.

2 to 3 types of vegetables to yield 1½ pounds (680 g), such as:

» Sweet potatoes, potatoes, or another root vegetable

» Yellow or red onions, bell peppers, or fennel bulbs

» Red cabbage, broccoli, or cauliflower

» Summer squash or zucchini

» Fresh corn, kernels sliced off the cobs

» Portobello mushroom caps or button mushrooms, trimmed

1 pound (454 g) extra-firm tofu or tempeh

1 tablespoon olive oil (OF: ¼ cup/60 ml broth)

2 tablespoons spice blend (see options on pages 221–247, such as Garam Masala or Fall & Winter All-Purpose Seasoning, or choose a store-bought blend)

Salt and black pepper

PINEAPPLE-BLACK BEAN BOWLS WITH ROASTED VEGGIES

MAKES: 2 large bowls // **TIME:** 15 minutes to prepare, 30 minutes to bake, not including time to cook beans and make Creamy Avocado-Lime Dressing

These simple roasted veggie and black bean bowls are inspired by Salsa's in Asheville, which serves food in lava stone bowls and giant wooden buckets. The vegan versions always have at least six different veggies, which is a nice touch, plus pineapple to make the dish really stand out. You could also add avocado (because that is never a bad idea).

2 sweet potatoes, cubed

One 10-ounce (284 g) bag frozen pineapple, thawed and juice reserved

2 red or yellow bell peppers, sliced into strips

1 yellow onion, sliced thin

1 tablespoon melted coconut oil (OF: ¼ cup/60 ml broth)

2 teaspoons ground cumin

Grated zest and juice of 2 limes

Salt and black pepper

2 cups (345 g) cooked black beans

¼ cup (60 ml) water

1 batch Creamy Avocado-Lime Dressing (page 151)

¼ cup (60 g) salsa

1 ounce (30 g) plantain chips (opt for the baked variety)

2 tablespoons pumpkin seeds

GF hot sauce, optional

1 Preheat the oven to 425°F (220°C). Line two baking sheets with parchment paper.

2 Place the sweet potatoes on one sheet and the pineapple, bell peppers, and onion on the other. Drizzle the sheets evenly with the oil, then sprinkle 1 teaspoon cumin and half the lime zest and juice over both trays. Season with salt and pepper.

3 Bake the sweet potatoes for 30 minutes, stirring halfway through, and the pineapple, bell peppers and onion for 20 minutes.

4 Meanwhile, heat the black beans in a medium saucepan over medium heat with the water, remaining 1 teaspoon cumin, and remaining lime zest and juice. Season with salt and pepper to taste.

5 Divide the sweet potatoes between two bowls, then top with the roasted vegetables and pineapple and the black beans.

6 Drizzle with the dressing, then top with the salsa, plantain chips, and pumpkin seeds. Serve with hot sauce if desired.

PINTO BEAN & GREENS ENCHILADA CASSEROLE

MAKES: 8 pieces // **TIME:** 10 minutes to prep, 30 minutes to cook, not including time to cook beans or make Cashew Queso

Authentic Mexican food isn't typically drowning in melted cheese. Lucky for us, it's actually quite easy to veganize. This quick casserole is our busy weeknight spin on a Mexican favorite, enchiladas. It combines all the flavors of enchiladas: smoky chipotle sauce, creamy (cashew) queso, and plenty of beans. We, of course, add plenty of vegetables for a more balanced meal that's easily customized; try swapping in different seasonings, beans, and greens, or substitute whole wheat tortillas or pitas for the corn tortillas.

1 Preheat the oven to 400°F (200°C). Coat a 9 x 13-inch (23 x 33 cm) baking dish with the oil.

2 Layer in the onion, kale, taco seasoning, and beans. Season with salt and pepper. Pour half the salsa evenly over the beans. Layer on the tortillas. Top with the remaining salsa and the cashew queso.

3 Cover with an inverted baking sheet and bake, about 30 minutes, or until the vegetables are soft and the salsa is bubbly.

4 Remove from the oven and let rest for 10 minutes. Slice and serve with the avocado, olives, and cilantro, if desired.

1 teaspoon olive oil (OF: omit)

1 yellow onion, diced

1 bunch kale, stemmed and chopped

2 teaspoons Taco Seasoning (page 226)

3 cups (510 g) cooked pinto beans, or two 15-ounce (425 g) cans pinto beans, drained and rinsed

Salt and black pepper

One 16-ounce (454 g) jar GF salsa (any variety)

12 corn tortillas

½ cup (80 g) Cashew Queso (page 237), or more to taste

Diced avocado, optional

Sliced black olives, optional

Chopped cilantro, optional

BLUEPRINT: A GRAIN, A GREEN & A BEAN

MAKES: 1 large bowl // **TIME:** 20 minutes to 1 hour, depending on the grain you choose, not including time to cook beans

A Grain, a Green & a Bean (aka The World's Most Perfect Vegan Meal) is the base for many a No Meat Athlete meal. With its endless variations (see table, page 99), it's the king of cheap, healthy, easy, and satisfying meals. Grains and beans are quite inexpensive if you choose wisely and buy them in bulk. The greens will cost more, but even a little goes a long way toward contributing plenty of flavor, color, and textural contrast (not to mention key nutrients). The "greens" don't even have to be green. You can add any vegetable—cooked or raw—that you have on hand.

Dress it up with any flavor combo imaginable, or dress it down with just salt and pepper. Take it further by sautéing an onion or pepper and garlic in the pot before you cook the grain for added depth. You can use dried beans that you've prepared, or even toss quick-cooking lentils into the pot with the grain as it cooks.

A Grain (see table; quinoa and brown rice are favorites)

Sea salt

A Green (see table; collards and kale, packed with nutrients, are our top picks)

A Bean (see table; cooked, unless using quick-cooking lentils)

A Spice Blend (see table) or other flavoring, such as hot sauce, salsa, vinegar, or tamari, to taste

In a large pot, cook the grain of your choice in the appropriate amount of water (according to the package directions) with a little salt. Once it's almost done, add the greens of your choice. While the greens wilt or soften, add the cooked beans or legumes of your choice. Then dress it up with more salt and a spice blend or whatever flavoring you're in the mood for.

FF: *For meals in minutes, choose prewashed greens in clamshell packaging or frozen greens; canned beans (drain and rinse before heating); and heat-and-eat grains.*

SF: *Make your beans and grains from scratch. If you have leftover grains and beans, freeze individual portions to make future meals come together in minutes.*

Here are some of our favorite flavors and ingredients:

A GRAIN
(½ cup)

Barley (100 g)

Brown rice (90 g)

Farro (105 g)

Millet (100 g)

Polenta
(coarse cornmeal; 70 g)

Quinoa (95 g)

Wheat or spelt berries
(95 g)

A GREEN
(2 cups chopped)

Broccoli (180 g)

Cabbage (napa, savoy,
green, or red; 140 g)

Collards (70 g)

Kale (30 g)

Spinach (80 g)

Swiss chard (70 g)

Zucchini noodles (220 g)

A BEAN
(1 cup cooked)

Adzuki beans (230 g)

Black beans (170 g)

Black-eyed peas (165 g)

Chickpeas (165 g)

Lentils (200 g)

Pinto beans (170 g)

Red kidney beans (175 g)

A SPICE BLEND

Fall & Winter All-
Purpose Seasoning
(page 229)

Fresh dill and tarragon

Garam Masala
(page 223)

Harissa (page 227)

Italian Spices
(page 224)

Jerk Spices (page 225)

Taco Seasoning
(page 226)

8 GREENS
You're Probably Not Eating

We all know the importance of getting our greens, but it's easy to reach for the same ones over and over (ahem, spinach and kale). Instead of relying on just one or two varieties, diversify your repertoire to make sure you're getting a good micronutrient balance. Here are some of the greens we turn to when we're looking to shake up our routine.

ARUGULA

Spicy and intense, arugula is not a green that blends into the background. This peppery cruciferous veggie is packed with vitamin A and folate, and it can be eaten cooked or raw. Toss on pizzas, puree into pesto, or sauté with garlic, then top with fresh peaches, walnuts, and lemon zest and juice.

Try spreading Spanish Red Pepper Spread (page 246) on a toasted baguette with arugula and lemon juice.

COLLARD GREENS

Known for their cholesterol-lowering, cancer-fighting properties, collard greens are sturdy, versatile greens rich in vitamins A, C, and K; they also supply a good dose of calcium. Sauté them with onions and garlic, then simmer in vegetable broth until tender. Or remove the stem from a large leaf, lightly steam it, and use it to wrap tacos, burritos, and sandwiches.

Try wrapping a Spicy Black Bean & Beet Burger (page 108) in a collard leaf along with some sliced red onion.

DANDELION GREENS:

Dandelion greens (yes, like the weeds in your yard) are peppery and bitter; they're also a good source of calcium, iron, potassium, and zinc, plus B vitamins and vitamins A, C, and D. Unlike spinach and chard, dandelion greens are somewhat low in the oxalic acid that can interfere with your body's ability to absorb calcium. They've also been used traditionally as an herb to support healthy liver function, and they are a natural diuretic, so they're great for reducing bloat after a race or travel. (Note: Don't actually pick the ones from your yard. Grow them from organic seed in your garden, or purchase them at the supermarket.)

Try making the base of your salads one part bitter greens, such as dandelion, and one part milder lettuce, such as romaine or green leaf. Bitter greens typically contain more nutrients than milder ones, but they can also be a bit overpowering on their own when eaten raw.

MÂCHE:

Also called lamb's lettuce, mâche is a fantastic plant-based source of omega-3 fatty acids. Deep green and velvety with a tender, nutty flavor, it's best mixed with other greens in salads.

Try adding mâche to a salad drizzled with Blueberry-Walnut Vinaigrette (page 155).

MIZUNA:

High in vitamin C, this mild Japanese mustard green is often found in baby green mixes. This feathery, frilly green also comes in a reddish-purple variety, and both have a mild peppery flavor that's a cross between kale and arugula. Use it raw in salads, or chop it and stir into any soup, stew, or tofu scramble.

Try stuffing it into a wrap with Tempeh Breakfast Sausage (page 63) and Miso Gravy (page 231).

NETTLES:

The nettles that sting you on the trail are actually a superfood. Each cup contains 7 calories, 2 grams of protein, and 6 grams of dietary fiber and provides 8 percent of your daily iron (two times what spinach boasts) and 42 percent of your calcium. Nettles are low in oxalates, compounds that inhibit the body from absorbing certain nutrients, so you can really access that calcium! Plus, they contain vitamin C, which helps you absorb iron. The sting goes away once you cook them, so wear gloves to handle them, then prepare them as you would spinach or kale. (Find them at co-ops and farmers markets in spring.) Toss with pasta, lemon juice and zest, and Cashew Cream (page 236) for a delicious carb-loading meal.

Try stirring chopped nettles into Anti-Inflammatory Miso Soup (page 112).

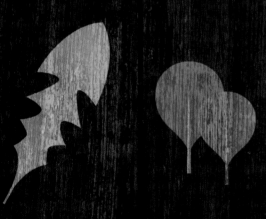
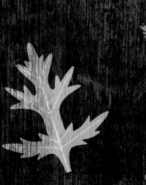
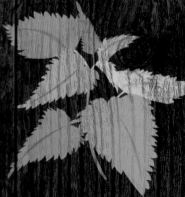

RAINBOW CHARD:

Part of the same family as beets and quinoa, Swiss chard is almost two veggies in one. Rainbow chard contains a unique set of phytonutrients and antioxidants, thanks to its multicolored stems and veins; it's also loaded with vitamins A, C, and K, plus magnesium. Remove the leaves from the stems and use as you would spinach. Sauté the stems with onions in soups and stews, or stuff them with hummus or nut butter for a colorful snack. (Note: Swiss chard contains high amounts of oxalic acid, which blocks nutrient absorption. However, steaming chard does help reduce its oxalic acid content.)

Try swapping chard for the cabbage in Colcannon (page 164).

TURNIP GREENS:

A calcium superhero, these potent greens contain almost 20 percent of your daily value per cup—in fact, their trademark bitter taste is due to the high calcium content. Prepare them as you would collard greens, or swap them for kale in any cooked recipe. Cooking them with onions, garlic, or spices helps tone down the bitterness without sacrificing nutrition.

Try substituting turnip greens for the collard greens in Caribbean Coconut Collards & Sweet Potatoes (page 122).

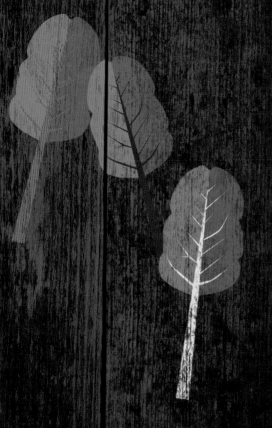

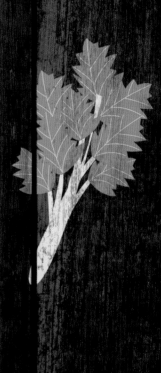

WHY SOAK GRAINS AND LEGUMES?

Grains and legumes contain varying levels of phytates, which interfere with your body's ability to access the nutrition in these foods. Soaking them overnight in water with a bit of acid can help remove some of the phytates and cut down on cooking time. It's a step that, once you do it a couple of times, becomes second nature. Every night when closing down the kitchen (washing dinner dishes and prepping tomorrow's daytime meals and snacks), glance at your meal plan and soak whatever bean or grain is on your list for the following day. (There are rare exceptions to this, such as sushi rice, which should not be soaked.) It only takes a minute, and the health benefits and time saved are worth the minimal effort.

Here's how: Add your legumes or grains to a large bowl and cover with water by at least 2 inches (5 cm). (You can add boiling water to further speed up the soaking process, but it's not necessary.) Add a splash of white vinegar. Give it a stir to prevent clumping and set aside. Before cooking, drain and rinse until there is no more foam. (The vinegar will not be detectable after you rinse.) Cook as usual, though soaked grains might cook faster, so keep a close eye on them.

WHY RINSE QUINOA?

Quinoa is coated with bitter saponins, which, while not harmful, can add a slightly unpleasant taste. We prefer to take the extra step to soak quinoa for at least a few hours, then rinse until the water runs clear and drain well.

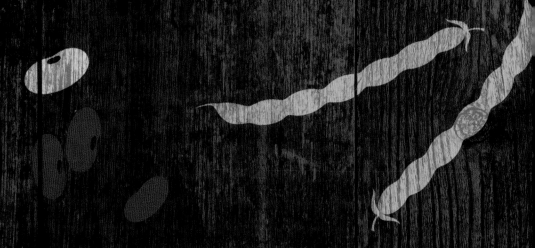

11 WAYS TO SPICE UP A GRAIN, A GREEN & A BEAN:

1 **CREAMY SALSA:** Top with salsa and hummus, preferably a roasted red pepper variety.

2 **COCONUT-LIME-CILANTRO:** Stir 1 to 2 tablespoons full-fat coconut milk into your bowl, squeeze the juice of ½ lime on top, then sprinkle with cilantro.

3 **SESAME-TAMARI-GINGER:** Grate ginger to taste onto each serving (start with ¼ teaspoon), along with a sprinkle of sesame seeds and a drizzle each of tamari and toasted sesame oil (OF: tahini thinned with water).

4 **LEMON-CAPER:** Add the juice of ½ lemon, 1 teaspoon olive oil (OF: ¼ mashed avocado), and 1 teaspoon chopped capers.

5 **SMOKY AND CHEESY:** Add a dollop of hummus, 2 tablespoons nutritional yeast, and a few hearty shakes of smoked paprika.

6 **ITALIAN STYLE:** Add dried oregano and basil to your bowl, then top with tomato-basil sauce.

7 **FRENCH VINAIGRETTE:** Drizzle your favorite vinaigrette (or our Classic French Vinaigrette; page 153) over hot or cold dishes.

8 **TABBOULEH STYLE:** Another hot or cold option. Toss with plenty of chopped flat-leaf parsley, lemon juice, and olive oil (OF: skip), as well as diced red onion and tomatoes.

9 **FRUIT AND NUTS:** Cook with 1 teaspoon each dried rosemary and thyme. Stir in dried cranberries or raisins and top with walnut pieces or pecans. (You can also add 1 teaspoon curry powder.)

10 **PESTO:** Top each serving with homemade or store-bought pesto, such as the ones on pages 233–235.

11 **OTHER FLAVOR BOOSTS:** See Chapter 8 for more options!

PEANUT BUTTER TEMPEH

SERVES: 2 to 4 // **TIME:** 10 minutes to prep, 30 minutes to bake

Rosetta's Kitchen in Asheville makes a peanut butter tofu that's delightful; however, it's cooked in oil before getting slathered in sauce, so it's not exactly ideal training fuel (but what a postrace feast it is!). Through quite a bit of trial and error, we created this lightened-up, slightly spicy tempeh version. Lightly steaming the tempeh reduces its bitterness. This dish is excellent with our Korean Tahini BBQ Sauce (page 230). Serve over mashed potatoes and steamed kale, or in a pita (gluten-free if necessary) with roast vegetables.

Two 8-ounce (227 g) packages tempeh, lightly steamed if desired

½ cup (130 g) natural peanut butter (creamy or crunchy)

⅓ cup (20 g) nutritional yeast

1 tablespoon fresh lemon juice or apple cider vinegar

1 tablespoon reduced-sodium, GF tamari

½ teaspoon black pepper

¼ teaspoon salt

⅛ teaspoon cayenne pepper or ¼ teaspoon crushed red pepper

⅓ to ½ cup (80 to 120 ml) warm water

1 Preheat the oven to 375°F (190°C). Line a baking sheet with parchment paper.

2 Slice each block of tempeh into 8 pieces. Smash each one slightly with the heel of your hand to increase the surface area.

3 In a shallow dish, combine the peanut butter, nutritional yeast, lemon juice, tamari, pepper, salt, and cayenne with enough water to form a thick sauce. The sauce should be lighter in color than peanut butter and be thinner than ketchup. If it's too thick, add water, 1 tablespoon at a time. If it gets too thin, whisk in another tablespoon or two of peanut butter.

4 Coat each piece of tempeh with the sauce and place on the prepared baking sheet. Spoon any remaining sauce on top of the tempeh slices.

5 Bake for 15 minutes, flip the tempeh, if desired, then bake for another 15 minutes, or until the sauce has formed a crust on the tempeh and turned medium brown. Serve.

Variation: For Peanut Butter Tofu, toss 1 pound (454 g) cubed extra-firm tofu with 1 tablespoon arrowroot powder, then proceed with the recipe as indicated.

NAKED SAMOSA BURGERS

MAKES: 12 burgers // **TIME:** 15 minutes to prep, 1 hour to cook

Prefer the filling of a samosa to its greasy, deep-fried wrapper? Then you'll appreciate these burgers. Though these are great on their own, they're not bean-based, so you could pair them with red lentils simmered with Garam Masala (page 223) and a little coconut milk for a more substantial meal.

1 Preheat the oven to 425°F (220°C). Line a baking sheet with parchment paper.

2 Boil or steam the potatoes in a large pot over medium-high heat until fork-tender, about 15 minutes. (We don't chop them, as cooking potatoes whole retains more of their potassium.) Drain and set aside.

3 Add the oil to the now-empty pot. Turn the heat to medium and add the onion, jalapeño, ginger, and garlic. Cook, stirring often, until the onions are soft, about 3 minutes. Add the garam masala, cumin, coriander, ½ teaspoon salt, the pepper, and turmeric and cook another 2 minutes, stirring often.

4 Place the potatoes in a large bowl. Using your hands or a potato masher, mash into bite-size pieces. Stir in the onion mixture, then fold in the peas, being careful not to mash the peas.

5 Using wet hands, form the mixture into 12 patties. Place on the prepared baking sheet and sprinkle with the remaining ¼ teaspoon salt. Bake the burgers for 30 minutes, flipping halfway through. Let cool for 5 minutes, then serve.

2 pounds (900 g) waxy potatoes, such as Yukon Gold

1 tablespoon olive oil (OF: 2 tablespoons broth)

1 large yellow onion, chopped

1 jalapeño, minced (seeds and ribs removed for less heat)

1-inch (2.5 cm) piece ginger, grated (see Tip)

2 garlic cloves, minced

1 tablespoon Garam Masala (page 223) or store-bought

1 tablespoon ground cumin

1 teaspoon ground coriander

¾ teaspoon salt

¼ teaspoon black pepper

¼ teaspoon ground turmeric

1½ cups (200 g) frozen peas, rinsed under cold water until slightly thawed

Tip: We use ginger frequently, so this hack has saved a lot of time. Scrub organic ginger well, using a paring knife to trim any particularly gnarly spots. Then use the back of a teaspoon to scrape off the rest of the peel. Chop roughly and process in a high-speed blender with about ¼ cup (60 ml) water per thumb-size knob of ginger until totally liquefied. Strain and freeze in an ice-cube tray. Once frozen, pop the ginger cubes into an airtight container. Voilà! Each cube is about 1 tablespoon. (This blender trick also works for garlic, fresh herbs, and peeled fresh turmeric—just skip the straining step.)

THANKSGIVING BURGERS

MAKES: 8 burgers // **TIME:** 15 minutes to prep, 30 minutes to cook, not including time to cook beans

These burgers are great for using up leftover fall vegetables, and they taste like Thanksgiving. They're also a low-fuss burger: Just mix and mash, bake, and eat. Lightly steaming the tempeh reduces its bitterness.

One 8-ounce (227 g) package tempeh, roughly chopped and lightly steamed if desired

1½ cups (270 g) cooked white beans

1 cup (205 g) roasted butternut squash cubes

1 cup (90 g) shredded raw or thawed frozen brussels sprouts

½ small yellow onion, diced

½ cup (60 g) chopped toasted pecans

¼ cup (30 g) dried cranberries

1 tablespoon Fall & Winter All-Purpose Seasoning (page 229)

Salt and black pepper

8 whole-grain hamburger buns

OPTIONAL TOPPINGS:

Quick Pickled Onions (page 240)

Lettuce

Whole-grain mustard

Prepared cranberry sauce

① Preheat the oven to 400°F (200°C). Line a baking sheet with parchment paper.

② Combine the tempeh, beans, squash, brussels sprouts, onion, pecans, cranberries, and seasoning blend in a food processor. Pulse a few times, season with salt and pepper, and continue to pulse until thoroughly combined.

③ With wet hands, scoop baseball-size portions into balls, then flatten into patties. Place on prepared baking sheet.

④ Bake for 30 minutes, or until golden brown, flipping halfway. Serve each patty in a bun with toppings, if using, or wrap up for later. (The patties can be refrigerated for up to 3 days or frozen for up to 2 months. To freeze, layer cooled burgers between slices of parchment and store in an airtight container for up to 2 months.)

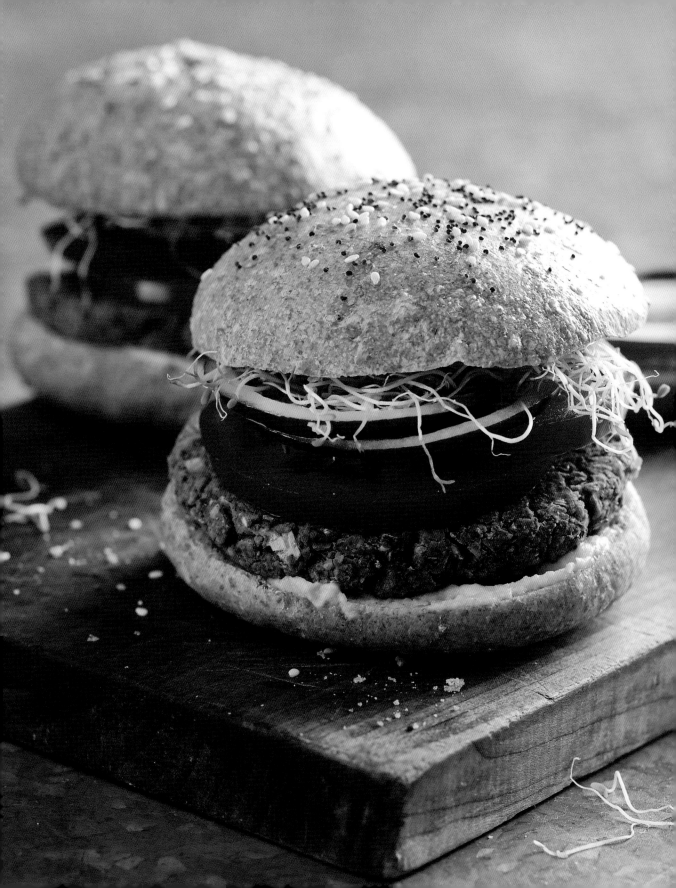

SPICY BLACK BEAN & BEET BURGERS

MAKES: 8 burgers // **TIME:** 20 minutes to prep, 40 minutes to bake

The go-to "meat" for a lot of veggie burgers is soy protein or vital wheat gluten. Instead, we opt for whole foods, namely beans, beets, and brown rice. The rice is the ingredient that binds the burgers and—along with the beets and beans—gives them a chewy, burger-like texture. Letting the finished burger mixture rest in the fridge for at least an hour will help them hold together better. If you're less concerned about that (or prefer to eat your burgers over greens and without a bun), then skip this step to save time. Serve with Sesame-Turmeric Oven Fries (page 173).

One 15-ounce (425 g) can black beans, drained and rinsed

1 cup (195 g) cooked brown rice

1 tablespoon olive oil (OF: ¼ cup/60 ml broth)

2 tablespoons Taco Seasoning (page 226) or Harissa (page 227)

1 beet, peeled and grated

1 carrot, peeled and grated

½ yellow onion, finely diced

2 tablespoons apple cider vinegar

2 tablespoons tomato paste

3 garlic cloves, minced

¼ teaspoon salt

Black pepper

8 hamburger buns

1. Preheat the oven to 400°F (200°C). Line a baking sheet with parchment paper.

2. Pulse the black beans and rice in a food processor until thoroughly combined. Transfer to a medium bowl and set aside.

3. Heat a medium skillet over medium heat, then add the oil. Add the taco seasoning and cook, stirring often, until fragrant, about 1 minute.

4. Add the beet, carrot, and onion and cook, stirring often, until the vegetables are soft, about 5 minutes.

5. Add the vinegar, tomato paste, and garlic and cook until the tomato paste has darkened and thickened, about 3 minutes. (There should be little excess moisture left in the pan. If there is, use a slotted spoon when transferring the vegetables in the next step to avoid soggy burgers.)

6. Remove from the heat and add the salt; season with plenty of pepper. Add the vegetable mixture to the bean-rice mixture. Stir (or mix with your hands) until thoroughly combined.

7. Using wet hands, scoop and mold the mixture into 8 patties, each about the size of a tennis ball. (If desired, refrigerate the uncooked patties for 1 hour or up to overnight. You can also freeze them for up to 3 months at this point and thaw them in the fridge overnight before baking.)

8 Place the burgers on the prepared baking sheet and bake for 30 minutes, then flip and cook for another 10 minutes. Let cool for 10 minutes on the baking sheet (the burgers will hold together better when they're not straight out of the oven).

9 Serve each patty on a bun with toppings, if using, or wrap up for later. (The cooked burgers can be refrigerated for up to 4 days.)

Variation: Use a cookie scoop to create 24 slider-size portions.

OPTIONAL TOPPINGS:

Quick Pickled Onions (page 240)

Lettuce

Tomato slices

Pickles or sauerkraut

You Won't Believe It's Cashew Ranch Dressing (page 152)

Whole-grain mustard

No-sugar-added ketchup

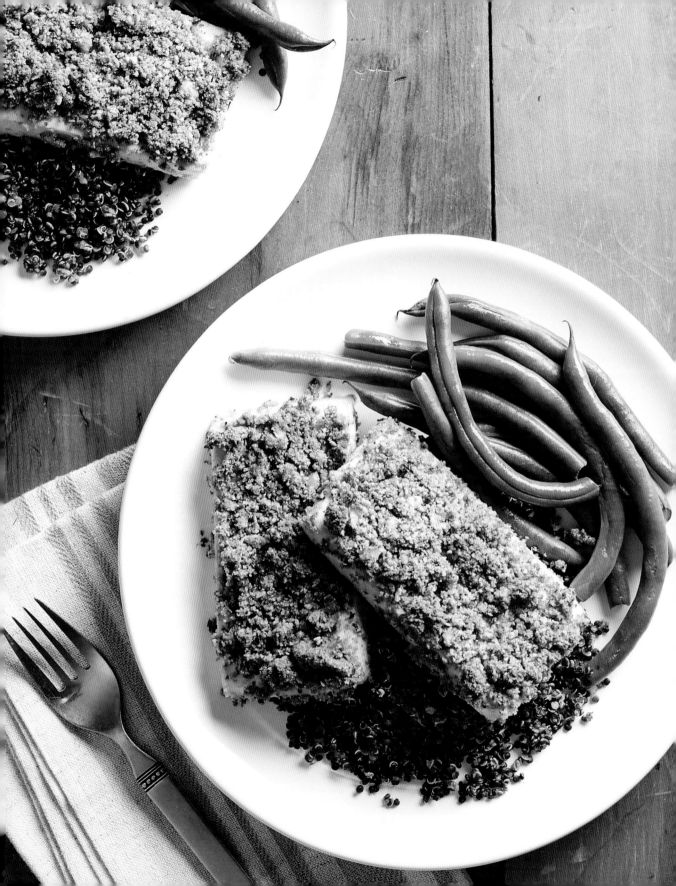

NUT-CRUSTED TOFU

MAKES: 8 slices // **TIME:** 10 minutes to prep, 20 minutes to cook

Trying to impress your dinner companion, but have very little time on your hands? This is the dish to make! Pistachios, tarragon, and lemon juice, plus a hint of Dijon mustard, turn a simple dinner into something special. Serve with steamed green beans (just call them *haricots verts* to keep the fancy facade going) and quinoa for a complete Parisian bistro-inspired meal. There's no need to press the tofu in this recipe; simply pat it dry. Any excess moisture will help the crust adhere to the tofu.

1 Preheat the oven to 375°F (190°C) and line a baking sheet with parchment paper.

2 Using a food processor (or a knife), chop the pistachios until they are about the size of the bread crumbs. In a pie plate, combine them with the bread crumbs, shallot, garlic, lemon zest, and tarragon. Season with salt and pepper.

3 Season the tofu with salt and pepper. In a small bowl, combine the mustard and lemon juice.

4 Spread the mustard mixture evenly over the top and sides of the tofu, then press each slice into the bread crumb mixture.

5 Place the tofu uncoated side down on the baking sheet. Sprinkle any leftover bread crumb mixture evenly on top of the slices. Bake until the tops are browned, about 20 minutes. Serve.

NOTE: *If you can only find salted pistachios, do not season the bread crumb mixture with salt in step 1.*

½ cup (70 g) roasted, shelled pistachios (see Note)

¼ cup (30 g) whole wheat bread crumbs, or GF if necessary

1 shallot, minced

1 garlic clove, minced

1 teaspoon grated lemon zest

½ teaspoon dried tarragon

Salt and black pepper

One 16-ounce (454 g) package sprouted or extra-firm tofu, drained and sliced lengthwise into 8 pieces

1 tablespoon Dijon mustard, GF if necessary

1 tablespoon lemon juice

ANTI-INFLAMMATORY MISO SOUP

SERVES: 4 to 6 // **TIME:** 15 minutes to prep, 30 minutes to cook

This soup is bursting with nutrition, with each ingredient specifically chosen for its health-supporting benefits. If you can't find dried mushrooms, swap in fresh, but add them with the onions. Turmeric is an anti-inflammatory powerhouse that supports everything from the liver and GI system to the joints, and the black pepper helps to maximize its absorption. We selected vegetables in an array of colors to provide a variety of antioxidants and phytochemicals.

1 tablespoon coconut oil (OF: ¼ cup/60 ml broth)

4 carrots, sliced into rounds

1 large yellow onion, chopped

1 ounce (30 g) dried shiitake mushrooms, broken or chopped into bite-size pieces

4 garlic cloves, minced

2 teaspoons ground turmeric

3 cups (720 ml) water

2 cups (480 ml) vegetable broth

½ cup (95 g) quinoa, rinsed and drained

¼ teaspoon black pepper

1 bunch bok choy, chopped

1 cup (70 g) finely chopped red cabbage

¼ cup (60 g) GF red miso

1 red or yellow bell pepper, chopped fine

3 scallions (white and light green parts), sliced thin

1 Place a large Dutch oven or heavy-bottomed pot over medium heat. Add the oil, then add the carrots and onion to the hot oil. Sauté, stirring often, until the vegetables are tender, about 5 minutes.

2 Add the mushrooms, garlic, and turmeric and stir to combine.

3 Add the water, broth, quinoa, and pepper, increase the heat to medium-high, cover, and allow to simmer for 15 minutes.

4 Add the bok choy and cabbage to the pot, reduce the heat to medium, and cover. Cook until the vegetables are slightly tender, about 3 minutes.

5 Remove the lid and whisk in the miso. Remove from the heat, add the bell pepper and scallions, and serve.

> **Tip:** Adding the miso at the end of the cooking process helps protect the delicate probiotics it contains.

"DON'T WASTE THE GOOD STUFF" SQUASH SOUP

SERVES: 4 to 6 // **TIME:** 15 minutes to prep, 30 minutes to cook, not including time to cook beans

Deborah Madison, one of the grandes dames of vegetarian cooking, has a cookbook called *Greens*, after the vegetarian restaurant she ran in the '70s. In the book, she shares a recipe for pumpkin broth that uses the stringy pulp and seeds of the pumpkin, along with the usual aromatics. This recipe got us thinking: Could we use our blender to create a pureed squash soup using the same technique? Turns out we could—and we did.

1 Preheat the oven to 425°F (220°C). Line a baking sheet with parchment paper.

2 Slice the squash in half. Remove the seeds and innards and transfer them to a large stockpot. Season the squash with salt and pepper and place cut side down on the baking sheet.

3 Bake the squash until fork-tender, about 25 minutes. Remove from the oven and flip the cut side up (to allow for faster cooling).

4 While the squash is baking, add the onion, carrots, celery, garlic, bay leaves, sage, thyme, rosemary, and water to the stock-pot with the squash innards and seeds. Bring to a boil, then reduce the heat to medium-low. Cook, uncovered, until the squash is finished baking. Remove from the heat and discard the bay leaves.

5 Scoop the squash flesh into a blender, then add the contents of the stockpot, plus the white beans. (You might need to do this in batches.) Puree until smooth, then return the soup to the stockpot.

6 Whisk in the miso, season with salt and pepper to taste, and serve.

Two 2-pound (900 g) butternut squash or 2 small pie pumpkins

Salt and black pepper

1 large yellow onion, peeled and quartered

2 carrots, roughly chopped

1 celery rib, roughly chopped

3 garlic cloves, chopped

2 bay leaves

2 tablespoons fresh sage, chopped

3 sprigs fresh thyme, leaves stripped and stems discarded

2 sprigs fresh rosemary, leaves stripped and chopped fine, stems discarded

6 cups (1.4 L) water

2 cups (360 g) cooked white beans

2 tablespoons GF mild white miso

GARLICKY ROSEMARY POTATO SOUP

SERVES: 4 to 6 // **TIME:** 15 minutes to prep, 35 minutes to cook, not including time to make Cashew Cream

Potato soup is pure comfort food, but the bulky main ingredient tends to dull any other flavor or seasonings. In addition to white beans for a nutrition boost, we add an aggressive amount of garlic and rosemary to ensure their flavors aren't muted. This soup reheats and freezes well.

1 tablespoon olive oil
  (OF: use ¼ cup/120 ml of the broth listed below)

1 large yellow onion, chopped fine

1 celery rib, chopped fine

8 garlic cloves, chopped

2 sprigs fresh rosemary, leaves stripped and minced

2 pounds (900 g) waxy potatoes, such as Yukon Gold, peeled and diced

One 15-ounce (425 g) can cannellini beans, drained and rinsed

1 bay leaf

¼ teaspoon black pepper, plus more to taste

4 cups (960 ml) vegetable broth

¼ cup (40 g) Cashew Cream (page 236)

¼ teaspoon salt

1 Place a medium stockpot over medium-high heat. Add the oil, then add the onion, celery, garlic, and rosemary. Cook, stirring often, for 5 minutes. Add the potatoes, beans, bay leaf, and ¼ teaspoon pepper and stir to combine. Add the broth, increase the heat to high, and bring to a boil.

2 Reduce the heat to medium-low, cover, and cook until the potatoes are tender, about 30 minutes. Remove from the heat and stir in the cashew cream. (If you prefer a smooth texture, puree half the soup in a blender.)

3 Add ¼ teaspoon salt and season with more pepper. Discard the bay leaf before serving.

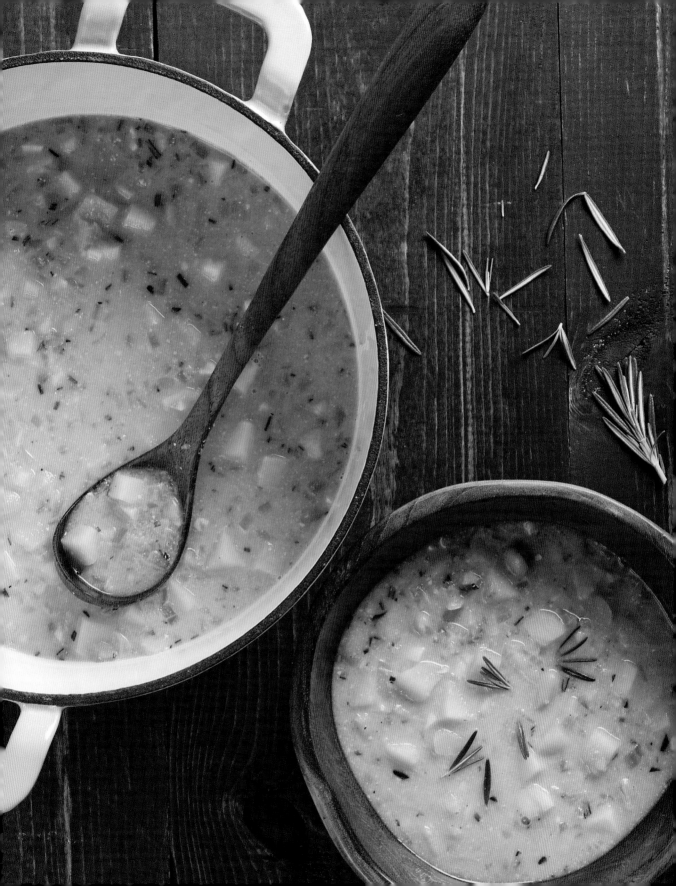

ALMOST INSTANT RAMEN

SERVES: 4 to 6 // **TIME:** 15 minutes to prep, 15 minutes to cook

Ramen has redeemed itself. Gone are the deep-fried noodles and MSG-laden flavor packets. Now, it's all about umami, veggies, and whole grain noodles. There are even versions that use brown rice or exotic varieties like purple or black rice! There's a whole world of healthier ramen out there these days, and it cooks almost as quickly as the originals. You can use any combo of veggies you like. We've also added instructions for turning this dish into a lunch "kit" (see Tip).

6 cups (1.4 L) vegetable broth

1 small yellow onion, diced

2 tablespoons wakame, optional

1 teaspoon minced or grated fresh ginger, or more to taste

1 teaspoon toasted sesame seeds

¼ teaspoon crushed red pepper, or more to taste

2 cups (140 g) broccoli florets

2 cups (140 g) shredded red cabbage

2 carrots, finely chopped

½ cup (115 g) kimchi

8 ounces (227 g) extra-firm tofu, cubed, or 1½ cups (345 g) cooked adzuki beans

Two 2.8-ounce (80 g) packages GF ramen or soba noodles

2 tablespoons GF red miso, or more to taste

2 nori sheets, cut into strips, optional

2 scallions (white and light green parts), sliced thin

Chopped cilantro

① Bring the broth to a boil in a large stockpot. Add the onion, wakame (if using), ginger, sesame seeds, and crushed red pepper.

② Reduce the heat to medium and add the broccoli, cabbage, carrots, kimchi, and tofu. Cook for 3 minutes.

③ Add the noodles, increase the heat to medium-high, and cook for 5 minutes or according to the package instructions.

④ Remove from the heat. Whisk in the miso and serve with the nori, scallions, and cilantro.

NOTE: *You can sub in any vegetables you like; try dried mushrooms, adzuki beans, or different kinds of seaweed.*

Tips:
To make lunch "kits," don't cook any ingredients before assembly. Divide the sesame seeds, ginger, crushed red pepper, wakame, vegetables, kimchi, and tofu into quart-size wide-mouth canning jars or glass storage containers along with the miso.

Pack the ramen noodles separately. The nori, scallions, and cilantro can be added to the jars or stored separately.

When ready to eat, bring water to a boil (use an electric kettle). Add the noodles to the jars, cover with boiling water, and put the lid on loosely. Allow to steep for 5 minutes, then stir and garnish.

You can freeze these kits for busy days. The texture is slightly altered and the miso's probiotics are rendered inert, but it's still a quick, healthy lunch.

ROASTED RED PEPPER MAC & CHEESE

SERVES: 4 to 6 // **TIME:** 25 minutes, not including time to make Roasted Red Pepper Queso

This lighter, veggie-infused version of mac and cheese is fast enough for a weeknight dinner, and it's a dish that'll have even the pickiest kids asking for seconds. It's ready in less than 30 minutes, even if you have to make the Roasted Red Pepper Queso from scratch. This is a saucy recipe—if you find there's too much sauce for your liking, save about one third of it for another meal, or stir in a pound of steamed broccoli or cauliflower. Serve with sautéed greens or steamed broccoli.

1 Steam or boil the squash in a medium saucepan over medium-high heat until tender, about 10 minutes.

2 Cook the pasta according to the package instructions.

3 While the pasta is cooking, add the squash to the roasted red pepper queso in the blender. Add cooking water from the pasta as needed, up to 1 cup (240 ml), until the mixture is pourable but still thick. (We used ⅔ cup/160 ml.)

4 Drain the pasta, reserving ½ cup (120 ml) cooking liquid.

5 Return the pasta to the pot and add the sauce. Stir to combine and heat over low until the sauce thickens and starts to bubble, about 5 minutes. If the sauce is too thick, add the reserved cooking liquid as needed. Serve.

FF: *Use canned butternut squash or cook a bag of frozen cubed squash.*

2 cups (280 g) cubed butternut squash (see Tips)

1 pound (454 g) small whole-grain pasta

1 batch Roasted Red Pepper Queso (page 237), prepared but left in blender and not heated

Tips:
The starches in raw butternut squash can cause a harmless but annoyingly itchy skin reaction in some people. If you have sensitive skin, wear gloves when handling raw squash.

Slice off the stem end. Take a small slice off the bottom of the squash to create a flat surface. Use a Y-peeler to remove the skin. After peeling, slice the squash in half. Scoop out the seeds and compost them or roast for a snack. Cube the squash and proceed with your recipe.

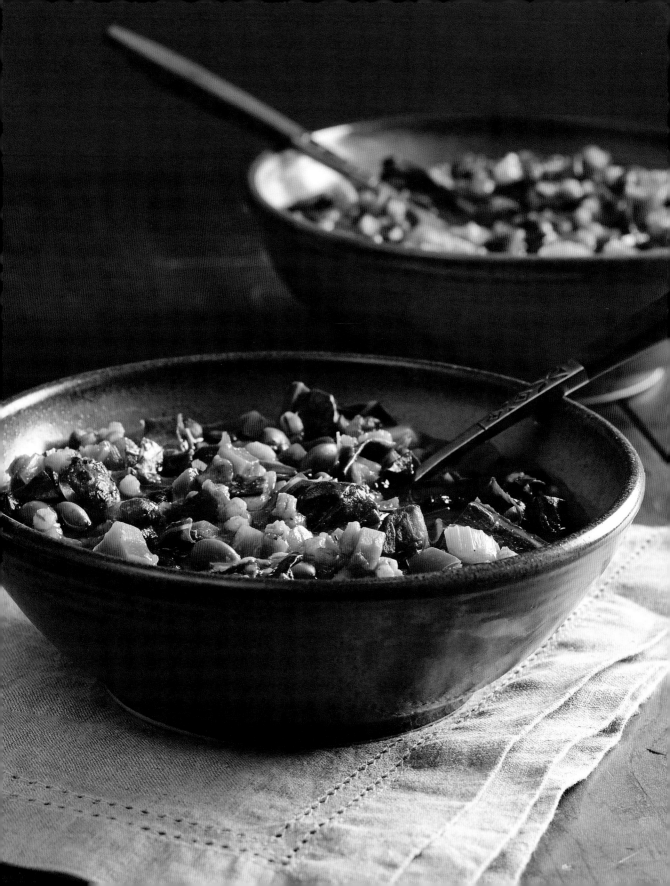

BLACK-EYED PEA & COLLARD STEW WITH SPICY TAHINI

SERVES: 4 to 6 // **TIME:** 20 minutes to prep, 40 minutes to cook, not including time to cook black-eyed peas

This dish was inspired by traditional New Year's Day ingredients and an Isa Chandra Moskowitz recipe. We start with a base of onion, carrots, and celery (mirepoix), layer in collards and black-eyed peas, then top it all off with a lightly spicy, smoky tahini sauce. You can add more or less Sriracha depending on your heat tolerance. While we like green bell pepper in this recipe, their unripe flavor and texture can sometimes be harsh. You can use a red, orange, or yellow pepper if you prefer.

① **To make the stew,** heat the oil in a Dutch oven over medium-high heat. Add the onion, bell pepper, carrots, and celery and stir to thoroughly coat. Cook for 2 minutes, reduce the heat to medium, and cover. Gently cook the vegetables for 5 minutes, stirring every minute or so. (OF: Keep adding broth as it evaporates.)

② Add the thyme, bay leaf, and cayenne, then the garlic. Stir and cook for 2 minutes.

③ Add the tomatoes with their juice, barley, and tamari. Cook, stirring often, until the moisture has evaporated, about 3 minutes.

④ Add the water, broth, and collards. Increase the heat to high, bring to a boil, then reduce the heat to medium-low. Cover and cook for 15 minutes.

⑤ Stir in the black-eyed peas. Remove from the heat and let sit for 15 minutes. Discard the bay leaf. Stir in the lemon juice and season with salt and pepper to taste.

⑥ While the stew is resting, **make the sauce.** Combine the nutritional yeast, Sriracha, lemon juice, maple syrup, liquid smoke, and tahini in a jar with a tight-fitting lid. (Adding other ingredients before the tahini prevents it from sticking to the bottom of the jar.) Add the water, 1 tablespoon at a time, shaking to mix, until the sauce is pourable but will stick to a spoon. Refrigerate until ready to serve.

Recipe and ingredients continue . . .

STEW

- 2 tablespoons olive oil (OF: ¼ cup/60 ml broth, plus more as needed)
- 1 large yellow onion, chopped
- 1 large green bell pepper, chopped
- 2 small carrots, chopped
- 1 large celery rib, chopped
- 1 teaspoon dried thyme
- 1 bay leaf
- ¼ teaspoon cayenne pepper or crushed red pepper
- 3 garlic cloves, minced
- One 14.5-ounce (411 g) can fire-roasted tomatoes with juice
- 1 cup (200 g) pearled barley, soaked (see Note)
- 1 teaspoon reduced-sodium tamari
- 2 cups (480 ml) water
- 1 cup (240 ml) vegetable broth
- 1 bunch collard greens, stemmed and chopped
- 2 cups (330 g) cooked black-eyed peas (if you use canned, go ahead and put in two 15-ounce/425 g cans; it's a very forgiving recipe)

1 tablespoon fresh lemon juice

Salt and black pepper

SPICY TAHINI

2 tablespoons nutritional yeast

1 to 2 tablespoons Sriracha sauce

1 teaspoon fresh lemon juice

1 teaspoon maple syrup

¼ teaspoon liquid smoke

¼ cup (60 g) tahini

¼ to ½ cup (60 to 120 ml) water

Sliced scallions

7 Top the stew with the sauce and scallions and serve.

NOTE: *If you don't want to soak your barley, that's fine; just rinse it well. Be sure to choose pearled barley for this recipe. It cooks faster because the bran has been partially removed. Pearled barley still contains plenty of fiber but is ready in far less time.*

> **Tip:** Want to use less salt? Add acid. How many times have you sat down to eat, taken your first bite, and then immediately reached for the salt to boost flavor? Instead of using salt, a healthier way to enhance flavor is by adding an acid, which is a common chef's trick. A drizzle of balsamic, splash of apple cider vinegar, or squeeze of lemon right at the end of cooking (or at the table) can help marry flavors and create contrast. And your blood pressure will thank you!

BASIC DAL

SERVES: 4 to 6 // **TIME:** 10 minutes to prep, 1 hour to cook, not including time to soak legumes

This stew of legumes and rice is about as simple as it gets, but it's incredibly comforting. It's easy on stomachs that are recovering from a hard day of exercise, and you can even eat it for breakfast! Feel free to add chutneys or Quick Pickled Onions (page 240) for even more flavor.

For most oil-free variations we typically "sauté" in broth, but here we want to draw out more of the flavor of the spices so we use coconut milk instead.

Cooking spices in fat helps release their volatile oils for more intense flavor—a process called "blooming." Using a bit of fat also helps your body to absorb more of the fat-soluble components in spices.

1 Place a large stockpot over medium heat. Melt the oil and add the ginger, garlic, jalapeño, cumin, and turmeric. Cook until the spices are fragrant, about 2 minutes.

2 Add the split peas and rice. Stir to combine, then add the broth. Increase the heat to medium-high, bring to a boil, then reduce the heat to low. Cook with the lid slightly ajar until the lentils and rice are tender, about 1 hour. (Add additional broth if you prefer a soup-like consistency.)

3 Season with salt and pepper, drizzle with lime juice and coconut oil, sprinkle with cilantro, and serve. (The dal can be refrigerated for up to 5 days.)

1 tablespoon coconut oil (OF: 1 tablespoon full-fat coconut milk solids), plus more for serving

1 tablespoon minced or grated fresh ginger

4 garlic cloves, minced

1 jalapeño, minced, seeds and ribs removed for less heat

½ teaspoon ground cumin

½ teaspoon ground turmeric

1 cup (200 g) yellow split peas or brown lentils, soaked overnight and drained

½ cup (200 g) brown basmati rice

4 cups (960 ml) vegetable broth or water, plus extra as needed

Salt and pepper

Fresh lime juice

Chopped cilantro

CARIBBEAN COCONUT COLLARDS & SWEET POTATOES

SERVES: 2 to 4 // **TIME:** 20 minutes to prep, 35 minutes to cook

Collard greens grow well in the South where we live; they're cheap at farmers markets and abundant in CSA shares. Once we learned of Callaloo-style collards, which hail from the Caribbean, this became a go-to recipe. To bulk it up, we added beans. Serve over rice if desired.

1 tablespoon coconut oil (OF: 1 tablespoon of the light or full-fat coconut milk listed below, plus broth as needed)

1 yellow onion, diced

3 garlic cloves, chopped

½ teaspoon crushed red pepper

2 bunches collard greens (about 2 pounds/900 g), stemmed, leaves chopped into 1-inch (2.5 cm) squares

1 large sweet potato, peeled and diced

One 15-ounce (425 g) can red kidney beans or chickpeas, drained and rinsed

One 14.5-ounce (411 g) can diced tomatoes with juice

1½ cups (360 ml) water (see Tip)

½ cup (120 ml) light or full-fat coconut milk

Salt and black pepper

1 Melt the oil in a large, deep skillet over medium heat. Add the onion, garlic, and crushed red pepper. Cook over medium heat for 3 minutes, then stir in the collards and sweet potato. Add the beans, tomatoes with their juice, water, and coconut milk.

2 Bring just to a boil, lower the heat to medium-low, and cook, covered, until the collards and sweet potato are tender, about 30 minutes.

3 Season with salt and pepper and serve.

> **Tip:** Don't waste the good stuff. Refill the tomato can, which holds about 1½ cups, and use that to measure the water needed for the recipe.

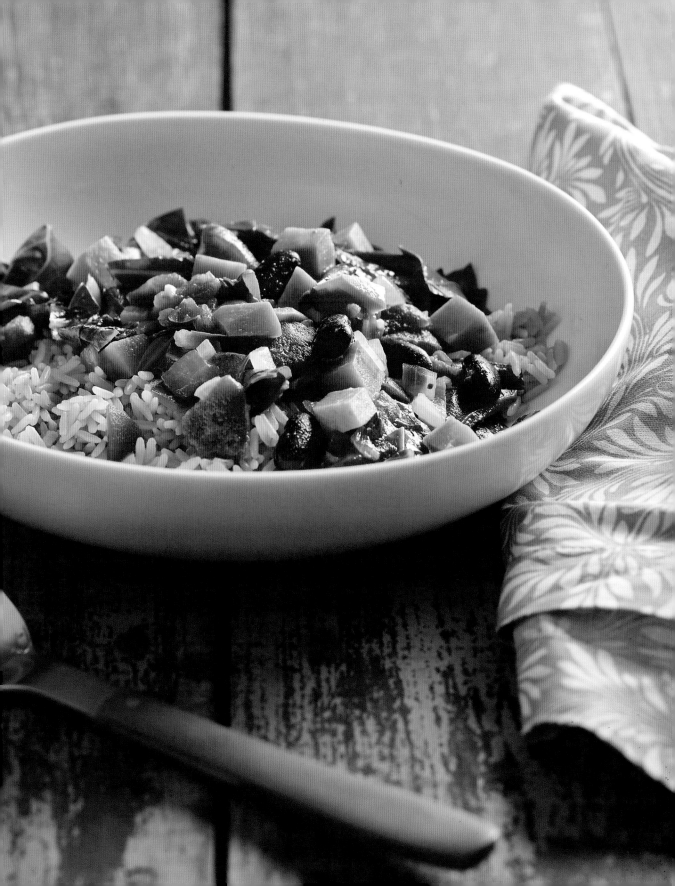

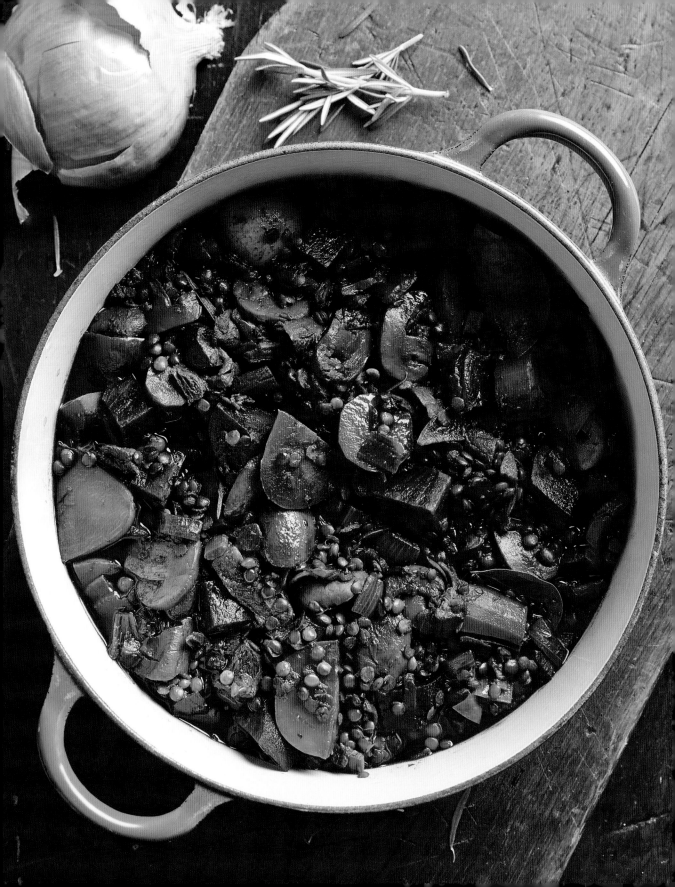

BEET BOURGUIGNON (BEET & LENTIL STEW)

SERVES: 4 to 6 // **TIME:** 20 minutes to prep, 45 minutes to cook, not including time to soak lentils

This stew is rich and hearty, ideal for a cold night after a long run. Inspired by the version in the *Green Kitchen Stories* blog, ours is simplified, and the lentils and beets play equally important roles; we've also added some miso for depth. A mix of red and brown or French lentils helps thicken the stew without adding flour or arrowroot powder. (Feel free to use all brown or French lentils if you don't have red, but using all red lentils will yield a mushy mess!) Be sure to chop all the veggies into rough 1-inch (2.5 cm) pieces.

1 Heat the oil in a large stockpot over medium heat. Add the onion and cook until it starts to soften and become fragrant, about 3 minutes. Add the mushrooms, celery, garlic, rosemary, thyme, and ½ teaspoon pepper. Cook until the mushrooms are dark and the vegetables are soft, about 5 minutes.

2 Add the tomato paste and cook, stirring constantly, until it darkens in color, about 2 minutes. Add the red wine and scrape the bottom of the pan to remove any cooked-on bits. Add the potatoes, beets, carrots, water, lentils, dried mushrooms, and bay leaves.

3 Increase the heat to medium-high and bring to a boil; as soon as it starts to boil, cover and reduce the heat to low. Cook until the vegetables are as tender as you desire and the lentils are cooked, about 30 minutes. Discard the bay leaves. Whisk in the miso and season with salt and more pepper to taste. Serve.

NOTE: *Save your clean, discarded mushroom stems for broth, or dehydrate and grind them for an instant flavor boost to broths and soups.*

1 tablespoon olive oil (OF: ¼ cup/60 ml broth)

1 yellow onion, chopped

One 10-ounce (283 g) package fresh cremini or white button mushrooms, trimmed and sliced (see Note)

2 celery ribs, chopped

3 garlic cloves, chopped

1 sprig rosemary

1 teaspoon dried thyme

½ teaspoon black pepper, plus more to taste

¼ cup (65 g) tomato paste

1 cup (240 ml) dry red wine

4 waxy potatoes, such as Yukon Gold, peeled and chopped

3 beets, chopped

3 carrots, chopped

3 cups (720 ml) water

1 cup (200 g) mixed lentils, soaked overnight, drained, and rinsed

1 ounce (30 g) dried mushrooms, broken into pieces

2 bay leaves

2 tablespoons GF red miso

Salt

FRENCH ONION STEW WITH MUSHROOMS

SERVES: 4 to 6 // **TIME:** 10 minutes prep, 1 hour 15 minutes to cook, not including time to cook beans or make Cashew Cream

Traditional French onion soup (*soupe à l'oignon*) employs a rich beef stock for depth; our plant-based version relies on two types of mushrooms and mushroom stock instead to provide meaty richness. We eliminate some of the hassle of caramelizing onions by letting the oven do the work. And we didn't forget the best part: Cashew Cream is spread thick on sourdough toast, broiled, then floated on each bowl. *Oui, oui!*

3 large yellow onions, sliced

One 10-ounce (283 g) package cremini mushrooms, trimmed and sliced

4 cups (960 ml) mushroom stock

6 sprigs fresh thyme

2 sprigs fresh rosemary, leaves stripped from stems and chopped fine

¼ teaspoon black pepper, plus more to taste

¼ cup (60 ml) red wine, such as Cabernet or Zinfandel

1 tablespoon arrowroot powder

3 cups (530 g) cooked cannellini beans or (690 g) cooked adzuki beans

1 ounce (30 g) dried mushrooms, broken into bite-size pieces

1 cup (240 ml) water

Salt

½ cup (80 g) Cashew Cream (page 236)

4 slices sourdough bread (GF: 4 slices GF bread)

1. Preheat the oven to 425°F (220°C).

2. Combine the onions, cremini mushrooms, 1 cup of the stock, thyme, rosemary, and ¼ teaspoon pepper in a large Dutch oven. Cover and cook in the oven for 1 hour, stirring and scraping down the sides of the pot every 20 minutes and adding the wine after 40 minutes.

2. Transfer the pot to the stovetop and place over medium-high heat. Preheat the broiler.

3. Carefully stir in the arrowroot powder, then add the beans, dried mushrooms, water, and remaining 3 cups stock. Bring to a low boil. Cook, stirring often, for 5 minutes. Remove from the heat and season with salt and pepper to taste.

4. Divide the cashew cream evenly among the slices of bread. Broil until the bread is toasted and the cashew cream is golden brown. Place a slice of bread atop individual bowls of stew and serve.

WRAPS & LEFTOVERS:
Quick Fuel for Everyday Activity

Most of us don't have the luxury of cooking a meal in the middle of the workday. That said, lunch is no time to give up on your commitment to good, healthy food or resign yourself to a PB&J or can of vegetable soup.

We're both fans of doubling up on meals in the evening, stashing leftovers for lunch the next day, then jazzing them up to ward off taste bud boredom. You'll notice throughout the book that we share tips on what to do with leftovers—and you should definitely think of them as intentional leftovers rather than some food that's been languishing in the fridge but you don't want to waste. Your lunch—or whatever meal you make with these extra helpings—should be worth looking forward to.

Five Ways to Make Last Night's Dinner
EVEN BETTER TODAY

1
WRAP IT UP.

Hearty appetites sometimes mean leftovers are in short supply, even if you intended to cook extra servings. If you're left with less than expected, that's OK. Use what remains of your stew, roasted veggies, or tempeh nuggets as a filling for a wrap, along with some greens and your favorite sauce.

2
MAKE A RICE BOWL.

Last night's Sheet-Pan Meal (see page 95) can be paired with raw veggies such as shredded carrots, cucumbers, or beets, plus a scoop of brown rice. Top with avocado or hummus, hot sauce or salsa, and lunch is a totally new meal.

3
CONSIDER YOUR CANVAS, AND GO BEYOND BREAD.

Simple staples like baked potatoes (sweet or regular), brown rice, quinoa, and even baked pita or tortilla chips can be the basis for dinner v2.0. If you used quinoa last night, use a pita today.

Bonus: Wrapping up last night's dinner could sway picky eaters, as Matt discovered with his son. On a plate? No way. But in a wrap and topped with Quick Pickled Onions (page 240)? The best thing ever!

4

ADD SOMETHING SPECIAL.

Do you ever have those moments when you're eating and you really wish you had a little something extra—think Miso Gravy (page 231), Quick Pickled Onions (page 240), or Cashew Cream (page 236)—to take your meal to the next level? Or midway through, you consider what it would taste like with hummus instead of salsa? Intentional leftovers mean you get a do-over, so do it!

5

GET YOUR GREENS.

When we think of wraps, most of us think of tortillas. But you can use lettuce or other leafy greens to make a portable salad of sorts for an extra dose of micronutrients and some variety. Try wrapping Peanut Butter Tempeh (page 104) in a steamed collard leaf (remove the stem) instead of a tortilla. Tuck cold Pinto Bean & Greens Enchilada Casserole (page 97) into romaine leaves with salsa. Toss cubed Nut-Crusted Tofu (page 111) with veggies and Classic French Vinaigrette (page 153), then stuff into butter lettuce leaves. If you aren't in the mood for finger food, use sautéed or steamed kale or collards, or mixed salad greens, as your base.

TWO WORKWEEKS' WORTH OF INTENTIONAL LEFTOVERS

- **MARINATED TOFU FETA** (page 238): Stuff in a pita with roasted red peppers, cucumbers, red onions, and chopped Kalamata olives.

- **JERK KIDNEY BEANS** (page 90): Add sautéed greens and turn it into a sub.

- **CHICKPEA QUICHE** (page 70): Slather on Cashew Cream (page 236), pile on arugula, and eat between two slices of toasted bread.

- **BREAKFAST HUMMUS** (page 56): Spread between two tortillas with onion and tomatoes for a "quesadilla."

- **SPICY ITALIAN BEAN BALLS** (page 81): Pile on a toasted baguette with Cashew Cream (page 236).

- **SAUCE FOR LENTIL-MUSHROOM NO-MEAT PASTA** (page 84). Add roasted peppers and eggplant, and sandwich between a whole grain Italian sub bun.

- **FARRO TABBOULEH** (page 182): Wrap in a whole wheat tortilla with white beans.

- **HARISSA BAKED TOFU** (page 71): Drain excess sauce and tuck into a whole grain pita with arugula. Serve the sauce on the side for dipping.

- **BAKED TEMPEH NUGGETS** (page 170) with Creamy Herbed Hemp Dressing (page 156): Add lettuce, tomato, and onions and stuff it into a wrap or pita.

- **FRENCH ONION STEW WITH MUSHROOMS** (page 126): Drain the broth and serve over toast, open-faced sandwich style, topped with Cashew Cream (page 236).

Chapter 5

GET YOUR GREENS: SALADS & DRESSINGS

While there's far more to a healthy, plant-based diet than salads, there's no doubt that we do eat a lot of them. A salad is a savory way to meet your veggie quota, and we strive to eat one almost daily. We look at them (as well as their sweet counterpart, smoothies) almost like a multivitamin, an insurance policy loaded with micronutrients and phytochemicals that protects you no matter what you decide to eat for the rest of the day. (Hey, cravings happen to us, too, now and then!) And it's very easy to cover most of the "Foods Worth Eating Every Single Day" (page 18) in your salad.

A big salad for lunch or as part of dinner can pack in leafy greens and cruciferous vegetables, onions, nuts or seeds (often in the form of dressing), sometimes fruit, and even beans as an easy protein topping. In addition to tasting great, salads deliver fresh, raw nutrition and a variety of textures and colors without a lot of effort.

Most of us have no trouble incorporating vegetables into our routine, but salads often get overlooked when you're looking to replenish major calories. After a hard workout, mealtimes usually focus on hot, cooked food. To combat this, one of the best tricks we've discovered is to prepare and serve your evening salad not right at mealtime, but right before you start cooking the rest of dinner, so that as everyone's hunger is stimulated by the smells from the kitchen, it's directed toward the ready-to-eat salad.

And of course, there's also Dr. Fuhrman's simple directive to "make salad the main dish." Since Fuhrman isn't addressing athletes specifically—some of whom will want more caloric density than a typical salad offers—our salads run the gamut from light and refreshing to hearty and filling. Some are meant to be served as sides, while others will fill you up even after a workout.

However you plan to eat your daily salad, don't negate all that good nutrition by topping your salad with store-bought dressings filled with oil, sugar, and salt. Drizzle on nutrient-dense homemade versions instead—you'll find lots of ideas in this section, most of them based on whole food fats from nuts or seeds, and healthy acids in the form of vinegars and citrus juice.

We hope you'll dive into this section and discover just how exciting greens can be—and in the process, firmly establish your "salad-a-day" habit!

STRAWBERRY-PISTACHIO SALAD

MAKES: 2 main course or 4 appetizer salads // **TIME:** 10 minutes,
not including time to cook grains or beans

Fruit is underutilized in salads, but we love the flavor, color, and texture strawberries provide. Grains and pistachios offer chewy and crunchy components to an otherwise delicate salad. Want to eat this for lunch all week? Keep the perishable ingredients (everything listed after the beans) separate, and build a fresh salad each day. You can use salted or unsalted pistachios. Celebrate the first bare-arms run of spring with this salad!

1 Combine the orange juice, lime juice, oil, ¼ teaspoon salt, and ⅛ teaspoon pepper in a large bowl. Toss the onions in the dressing; add the grains, strawberries, and beans and toss to combine.

2 Season with salt and pepper to taste. (At this point, the salad can be refrigerated until ready to serve, up to 1 day.)

3 Add the greens and cilantro and toss to combine. Sprinkle with the pistachios, top with the avocado, and drizzle with the vinegar. Serve.

¼ cup (60 ml) orange juice

2 tablespoons fresh lime juice

1 tablespoon olive oil (OF: omit)

¼ teaspoon salt, plus more to taste

⅛ teaspoon black pepper, plus more to taste

½ small red onion, chopped or sliced

2 cups (290 g) cooked grains, such as barley, cooled

2 cups (1 pint/290 g) strawberries, hulled and chopped

1½ cups (270 g) cooked cannellini beans, or one 15-ounce (425 g) can cannellini beans, drained and rinsed

One 5- to 6-ounce (140 to 170 g) container mixed baby greens

½ cup (30 g) chopped cilantro

½ cup (70 g) roasted, shelled pistachios, chopped

½ avocado, diced

High-quality balsamic vinegar

BLUEPRINT: CLASSIC KALE SALAD

MAKES: 2 main course or 4 appetizer salads // **TIME:** 20 minutes to prep, not including time to "marinate"

Kale salads are a staple for plant-based eaters, and these days you're as likely to find them on salad bars as you are on upscale restaurant menus. Kale stands up to big flavors and it is sturdy enough to survive a bit of mistreatment (e.g., being forgotten in the fridge for a few days).

There are really only two things you can do to mess up kale salad beyond repair: not removing the stems from the leaves, and not massaging the greens. Kale stems are unpleasant to eat raw and it's easy to remove them. And if you simply coat kale in dressing rather than massage it on, the dressing doesn't get a chance to soak in and tenderize the kale, so the leaves stay quite tough. (And a lesser grievance is giant pieces of kale—no one can gracefully shove half a kale leaf in their mouth!) This formula-style recipe breaks down the simplest of treatments for kale.

2 bunches kale, stemmed and chopped into bite-size pieces

2 tablespoons GF vinegar or citrus juice, plus more to taste

1 tablespoon olive oil (OF: omit)

½ teaspoon salt, plus more to taste

¼ teaspoon dried herbs or spices such as thyme or ground cumin, optional

2 cups (220 g) shredded or chopped mixed crunchy vegetables, such as bell peppers, beets, carrots, and celery

¼ cup (40 g) finely chopped red onion, or 2 scallions (white and light green parts), sliced

Black pepper

½ cup (70 g) seeds or chopped nuts

¼ cup (30 g) dried fruit

1 Place the kale in a large bowl and drizzle with the vinegar and oil, then add ½ teaspoon salt and the herb(s), if using. Use your hands to massage the kale thoroughly, until it starts to darken in color and look slick.

2 Add the mixed vegetables and onion and toss to combine. Refrigerate for 8 hours or overnight, until ready to serve.

3 Just before serving, season with salt, pepper, and vinegar to taste and sprinkle with the nuts and dried fruit. Serve immediately or refrigerate for up to 3 days.

Variation: For Rainbow Raw Salad, skip the kale and use a rainbow of other veggies instead:

» Beets, celery, carrots, and red cabbage with Lemon-Tahini Dressing (page 146)

» Fennel and bell peppers with Creamy Avocado-Lime Dressing (page 151; this will only last 1 day in the fridge due to the avocado)

» Cauliflower and bell peppers with Lemon-Thyme Dressing (page 149)

» Use the same technique to massage the vegetables to help them break down.

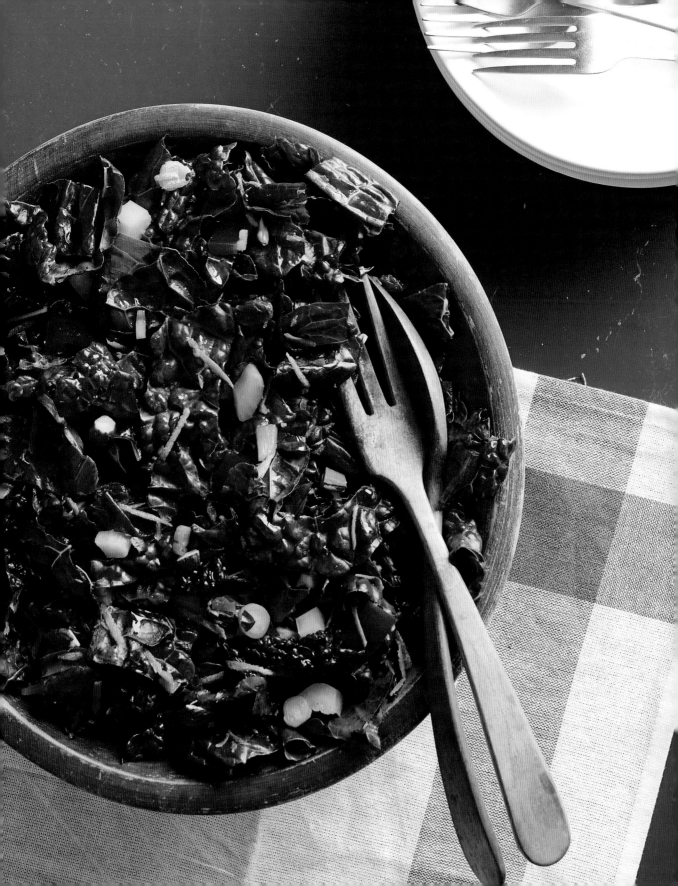

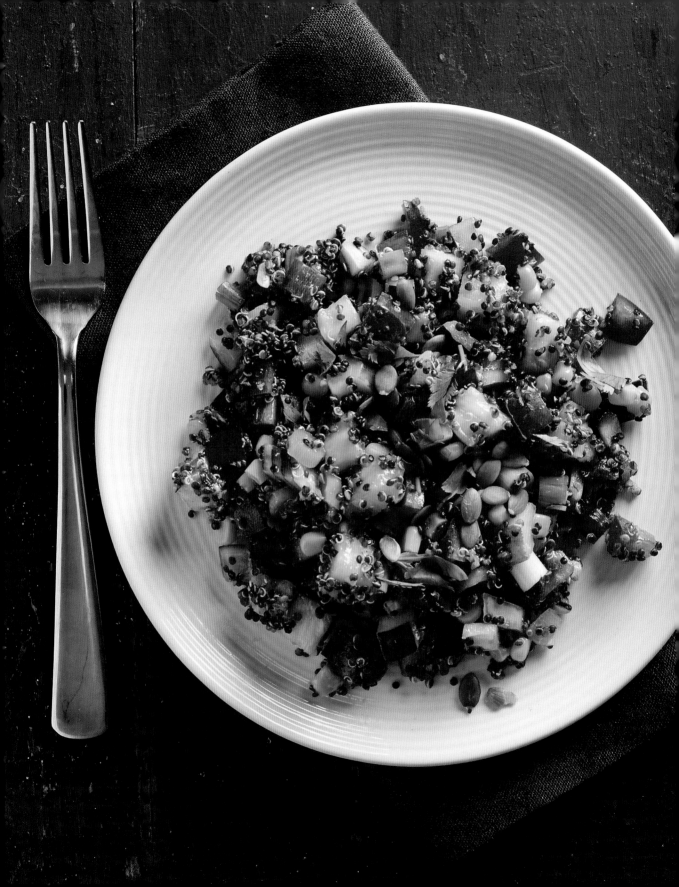

CONFETTI QUINOA SALAD

MAKES: 2 main course or 4 appetizer salads // **TIME:** 15 minutes,
not including time to cook quinoa or make dressing

Fun and festive, this quinoa salad involves a lot of chopping but not much work beyond that. Because there's nothing that can wilt, it holds up well, so add it to your brown-bag lunch rotation.

1 Combine the quinoa, pineapple, corn, bell pepper, red onion, scallions, and tomato in a large bowl. (If not eating immediately, keep the salad separate from the dressing. You need to use the Creamy Avocado-Lime dressing within 1 day, but the undressed salad will keep for up to 3 days.)

2 Toss with the dressing and season with salt and pepper. Garnish with the pumpkin seeds and cilantro and serve.

2 cups (370 g) cooked quinoa, cooled

1 cup (165 g) diced pineapple or mango, thawed if frozen

1 cup (165 g) corn kernels, thawed if frozen

1 large red or yellow bell pepper, diced

1 red onion, diced

2 scallions (white and light green parts), sliced

1 large tomato, chopped (about 1 cup/180 g)

1 batch Creamy Avocado-Lime Dressing (page 151) or Lime-Cumin Dressing (page 150)

Pinch of salt and black pepper

½ cup (80 g) pumpkin seeds, preferably raw and unsalted

¼ cup (15 g) chopped cilantro

WINTER SUNSHINE SALAD

MAKES: 2 main course or 4 appetizer salads // **TIME:** 15 minutes

When you're sick of winter and unable to take another bite of soup or stew, treat yourself to this salad. Crunchy and bursting with flavor, it's a welcome diversion from the heavy comfort food of winter. Thanks to the citrus and avocado, it dresses itself.

2 small fennel bulbs, cored and thinly sliced

2 ruby red grapefruits, supremed and juice reserved (see Tip)

2 cups (140 g) shredded red cabbage

1 red or orange bell pepper, thinly sliced

1 tablespoon fresh lime juice

Salt and black pepper

½ cup (30 g) chopped cilantro

1 avocado, diced or sliced

¼ cup (30 g) walnut pieces

1 Combine the fennel, grapefruit segments and juice, cabbage, bell pepper, and lime juice in a large bowl. Season with salt and pepper to taste, then toss to combine. (At this point, you can refrigerate the salad overnight.)

2 When ready to serve, add the cilantro and toss to combine. Divide into bowls, then divide avocado and walnuts evenly between salads.

Tip: The secret to peel-free citrus segments is a technique called supreming. To supreme citrus, slice off both ends just until the flesh is exposed. Starting at the top, use a paring knife to slice the rind and white pith off, removing as little flesh as possible. Hold the fruit in your nondominant hand and make shallow vertical slices between each segment, along the natural divisions. Do this over a bowl to catch any juices. Discard any seeds as well as the middle part and the membrane that separates the segments.

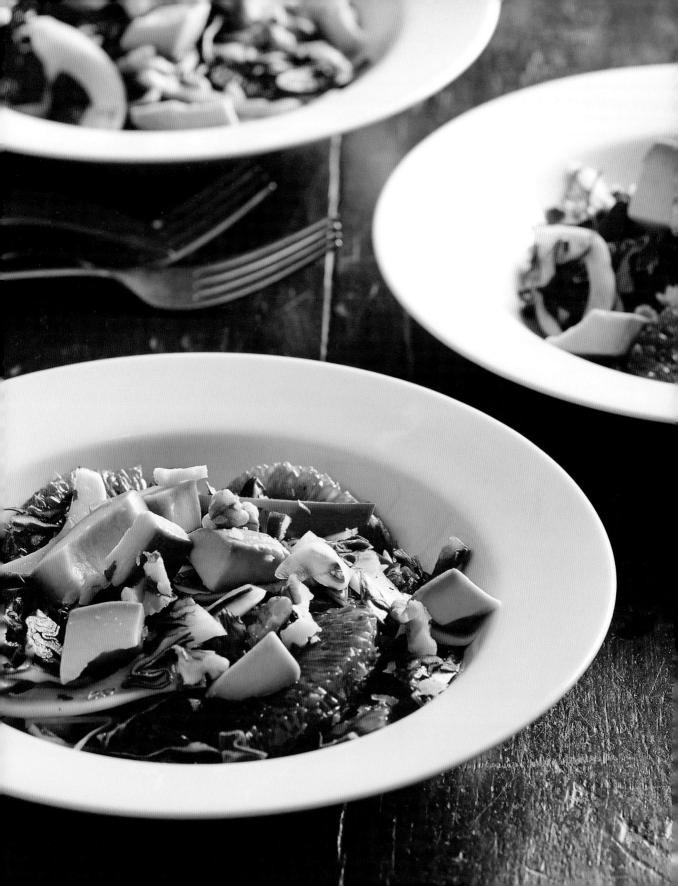

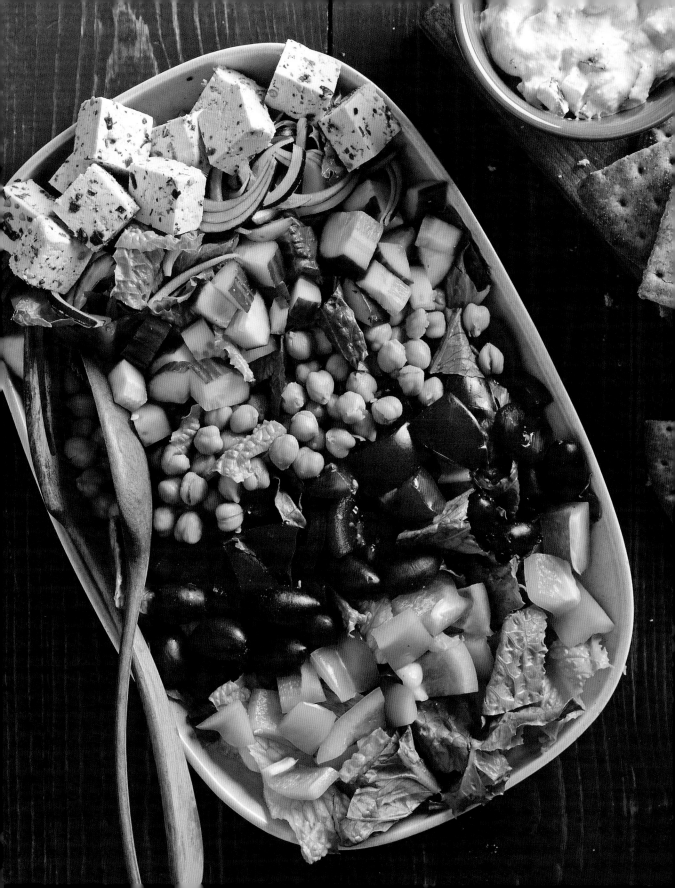

GREEK CHOPPED SALAD

MAKES: 2 main course or 4 appetizer salads // **TIME:** 55 minutes, not including time to make Marinated Tofu Feta and Cashew Tzatziki

Greek salads are ubiquitous on lunch menus, but without the feta you're left with a pile of veggies and an oily dressing. Here we've upgraded the vegetables, swapped the feta for a marinated, oil-free tofu, and added Cashew Tzatziki for a creamy, tangy contrast.

1 Place the lettuce in a large bowl. Arrange the bell pepper, tomato, chickpeas, cucumbers, olives, onion, and tofu feta on top. (We prefer rows.)

2 Drizzle with the cashew tzatziki, then arrange the pita around the edges. Serve with the lemon wedges.

2 romaine hearts, washed, dried, and chopped

1 red or yellow bell pepper, roasted or raw, chopped

1 large tomato, diced, or 1 cup (150 g) halved grape tomatoes

1 cup (165 g) cooked chickpeas

½ cup (50 g) chopped cucumber

½ cup (90 g) pitted Kalamata olives

¼ cup (40 g) chopped red onion

½ batch Marinated Tofu Feta (page 238), OF version

¼ cup plus 2 tablespoons (45 g) Cashew Tzatziki (page 239)

Whole grain pita wedges or pita chips

Lemon wedges

VIETNAMESE VEGGIE & RICE NOODLE SALAD

MAKES: 4 main course salads // **TIME:** 35 minutes to prepare, not including time to "pickle"

While requiring a bit of forethought, this refreshingly crunchy salad is more than worth it on a hot summer day. You can even skip cooking the tofu if you can't bear to turn on the stove. In lieu of a traditional dressing, we drizzle it with an avocado-ginger aïoli. Have leftovers? Stuff them into spring roll wrappers or collard leaves.

4 large carrots, grated

1 small daikon radish, peeled and grated

1 English cucumber, thinly sliced

¼ cup (60 ml) GF rice vinegar

1 tablespoon sugar

¼ teaspoon salt, plus more to taste

2 avocados, halved and pitted

1-inch (2.5 cm) piece ginger, peeled and minced

2 tablespoons to ¼ cup (60 ml) water

1 tablespoon fresh lime juice

1 garlic clove

1 tablespoon coconut oil (OF: omit)

One 16-ounce (454 g) package sprouted or extra-firm tofu, drained and cubed

Black pepper

8 ounces (227 g) brown rice noodles

2 cups (210 g) mung bean sprouts

½ cup (30 g) chopped cilantro or mint

Unsalted peanuts

Chili sauce, such as Sriracha sauce, optional

1 Combine the carrots, radish, cucumber, vinegar, sugar, and ¼ teaspoon salt in a small bowl. Refrigerate for 1 hour or up to 1 day.

2 Pulse the avocados, ginger, 2 tablespoons of the water, lime juice, and garlic in a blender until combined. Continue to process until the sauce has the consistency of aïoli, adding more water, 1 tablespoon at a time, if necessary (we used it all). Transfer to a container with a tight-fitting lid and set aside.

3 Heat a medium cast-iron skillet over medium-high heat. Add the oil to the pan.

4 Place the tofu in a single layer in the skillet. Cook until brown, about 8 to 10 minutes. Season with salt and pepper. Set aside to cool.

5 Prepare the rice noodles according to the package directions. Drain and rinse with cold water.

6 Toss the "pickled" vegetables with the noodles, then divide into bowls. Top with the tofu, bean sprouts, and cilantro. Drizzle with the avocado sauce. Garnish with the peanuts and chili sauce, if using, and serve. (Leftover salad ingredients can be refrigerated for up to 3 days; the dressing should be consumed within 1 day.)

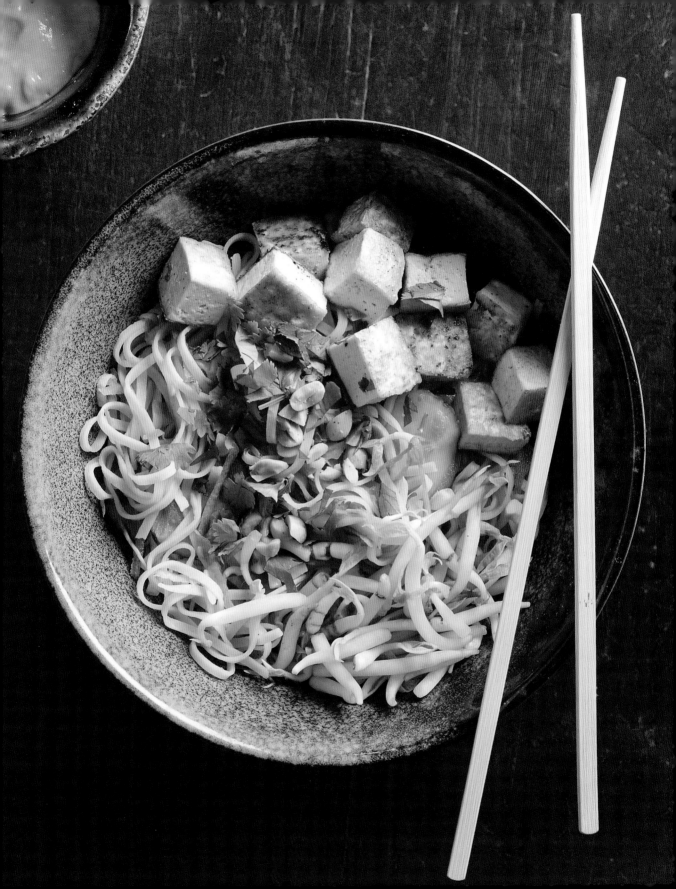

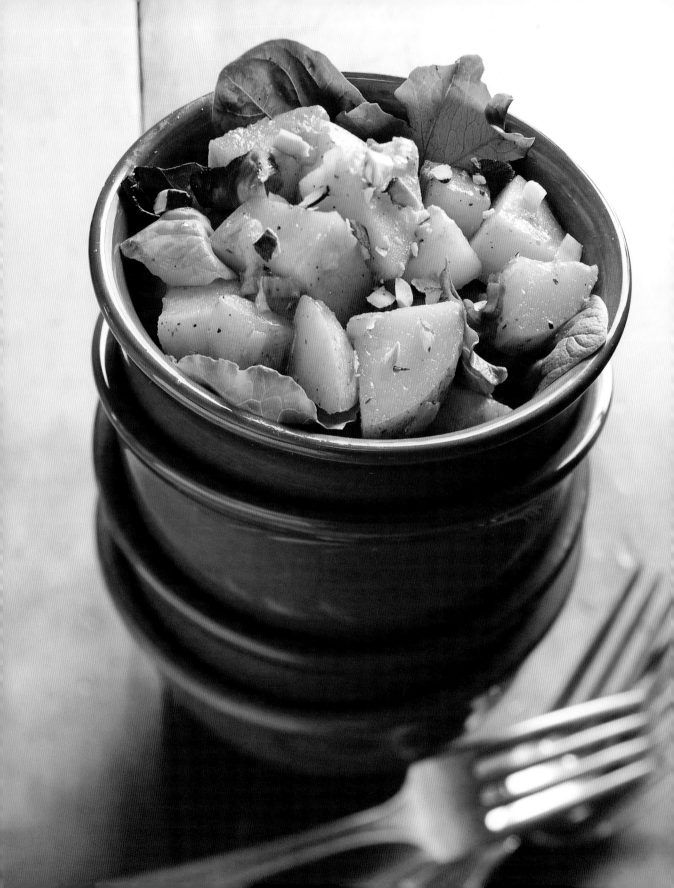

SMOKY POTATO SALAD OVER GREENS

SERVES: 4 to 6 // **TIME:** 25 minutes

Have no fear: This is not the goopy, neon-yellow, mayo-laden potato salad we all avoid at potlucks and picnics. First of all, there's no mayo. Secondly, there are greens, which accurately categorizes this as an actual salad. The dressing is smoky and vinegar-based and soaks right into the potatoes. It can be served warm or chilled. If desired, add 1 chopped red or yellow bell pepper before serving. Want more smokiness? Toss some Shiitake Bakin' (page 62) on top.

1 Steam or boil the potatoes in a large pot over medium-high heat until fork-tender, about 15 minutes. Drain and let cool in a single layer.

2 Meanwhile, whisk the vinegar, scallions, oil, maple syrup, tomato paste, mustard, salt, paprika, pepper, and liquid smoke together in a large bowl.

3 Chop the potatoes into bite-size pieces. Add to the bowl and toss gently with the dressing. Serve over the greens and top with almonds if serving immediately. The salad can be refrigerated for up to 5 days (though the oil-free version will only last a day due to the avocado), then combined with the greens and almonds before eating.

2 pounds (900 g) waxy potatoes, such as Yukon Gold

¼ cup (60 ml) apple cider vinegar

2 scallions (white and light green parts), sliced

2 tablespoons olive oil (OF: omit or use ½ avocado, mashed)

1 teaspoon maple syrup

1 teaspoon tomato paste

½ teaspoon GF Dijon mustard

½ teaspoon salt

½ teaspoon smoked paprika

¼ teaspoon black pepper

2 drops liquid smoke

12 ounces (340 g) baby greens

¼ cup (30 g) unsalted, roasted almonds, chopped

BLUEPRINT: HOMEMADE SALAD DRESSING

SERVES: 4, but easily scaled up // **TIME:** 5 minutes

Believe it or not, you really don't need a recipe for salad dressing. You can create endless varieties, with ingredients you probably already have on hand, if you stick to the ratios listed in this simple blueprint. And although you might never have considered oil-free dressing as a possibility, dressings that use alternative ingredients will actually bind better than traditional versions because straight oil doesn't mix well with other liquids (such as vinegar and citrus juice).

1 part acid (vinegar, tomatoes, citrus juice, or mustard)

3 parts oil or creamy ingredient (avocado, nut butter, tofu, hummus, or pureed beans)

Flavorings to taste (fresh or dried herbs, spices, onion/shallot, ginger, or garlic)

Salt and black pepper to taste

Process all the ingredients in a blender or shake together in a small jar with a lid until smooth. Dressings may thicken after being refrigerated, so add additional water as desired before serving. Refrigerate in an airtight container for up to 5 days.

Try these oil-free dressing ideas:

- Lime juice with silken tofu and basil

- Orange juice with avocado and cilantro

- Balsamic vinegar with cashew butter and rosemary

- Rice vinegar with tahini and ginger

- Dijon mustard with chickpeas, shallots, and tarragon

- Salsa with avocado and cumin

And for some more traditional, oil-based dressings, try:

- Red wine vinegar with olive oil and dried dill

- Apple cider vinegar with grapeseed oil and garlic

- Lemon juice with sesame oil and coriander

GREEN ON GREENS DRESSING

SERVES: 8 to 12 / Makes about 2 cups (480 ml) // **TIME:** 5 minutes

Serve this mild dressing, inspired by the house dressing at Angelica Kitchen in the East Village in New York City, atop cooked grains, on simple green salads, or as a dip. The parsley and scallion brighten up the tahini, while the sour and salty umeboshi paste (sour Japanese plum) and tangy apple cider vinegar are great for digestion. Tamari adds a salty richness. Why "Green on Greens"? Put it on a salad and you'll see!

Process all the ingredients in a blender until smooth. The dressing will thicken upon sitting, so add additional water as desired before serving. Refrigerate in an airtight container for up to 2 days.

NOTE: *With so few ingredients, making any substitutions will affect the outcome of this dressing. However, we know umeboshi may be one of the most "out there" ingredients we use in the book, so we tested this without the umeboshi, using 1½ teaspoons apple cider vinegar and ½ teaspoon tamari. The result? A pretty good substitute.*

¾ cup (180 ml) water, plus extra as needed

½ cup (30 g) chopped flat-leaf parsley

¼ cup (60 g) tahini

1 scallion (white and light green part), sliced

1 tablespoon apple cider vinegar

2 teaspoons umeboshi paste or 2 umeboshi plums, pitted and roughly chopped (see Note)

1 teaspoon reduced-sodium tamari

LEMON-TAHINI DRESSING

SERVES: 6 to 8 / Makes 1¼ cups (300 ml) // **TIME:** 5 minutes

Life before tahini-based salad dressings is a distant memory. Discovering this delightfully bitter, creamy ingredient caused traditional vinaigrettes to fall out of favor. This simple dressing gets most of its flavor from a careful balance of tahini, lemon, and salt; try it not only on salads but as a dip for raw vegetables, baked tofu, and tempeh nuggets. It also makes a surprisingly good pasta sauce, especially in spring and summer. Toss with linguine, bitter greens, halved grape tomatoes, and spring onions, then top with good flaky salt and nutritional yeast.

The dressing will thicken slightly after being refrigerated. If you're using it on a "wet" salad or massaged kale, keep it slightly thick. If you're tossing it with romaine or delicate baby greens, thin it out until pourable.

¼ cup (60 ml) fresh lemon juice (about 2 lemons)

1 teaspoon sugar or other sweetener (such as maple syrup or date)

1 small garlic clove, chopped

½ cup (120 g) GF tahini

¼ teaspoon salt

⅛ teaspoon black pepper

¼ to ½ cup (60 to 120 ml) water

Pulse the lemon juice, sugar, garlic, tahini, salt, and pepper in a high-speed blender to combine. Slowly add the water, starting with ¼ cup (60 ml), until it reaches the desired consistency. Refrigerate in an airtight container for up to 5 days.

MANGO-ORANGE DRESSING

SERVES: 6 to 8 / Makes about 1½ cups (360 ml) // **TIME:** 5 minutes

The trick to oil-free dressings is creating just the right balance of flavors. Here, we use three bright acids, some sweeter or stronger than others, paired with mango. Cilantro brightens it up, and the final dressing is sweet, tangy, and 100 percent oil-free. Serve on black beans, tofu, or any summer salad. If your mango is very ripe, you can omit the sugar.

Process the mango, orange juice, lime juice, rice vinegar, sugar, and salt in a blender until smooth. Stir in the cilantro. Refrigerate in an airtight container for up to 2 days.

1 cup (165 g) diced mango, thawed if frozen

½ cup (120 ml) orange juice

2 tablespoons fresh lime juice

2 tablespoons GF rice vinegar

1 teaspoon raw sugar, optional

¼ teaspoon salt

2 tablespoons chopped cilantro

ROASTED GARLIC DRESSING

SERVES: 4 to 6 / Makes about ⅔ cup (160 ml) // **TIME:** 5 minutes

Roasted garlic lends a creaminess to this dressing with absolutely no oil (or even any whole food fat, for that matter!). It pairs well with root vegetables, hearty raw greens like kale, and roasted veggies. It also works well as a marinade.

1 head roasted garlic, cloves removed from skins (see Tip)

3 tablespoons red wine or apple cider vinegar

1 tablespoon balsamic vinegar

1 teaspoon sugar or other sweetener (such as maple syrup or dates)

¼ teaspoon salt

⅛ teaspoon black pepper

¼ teaspoon dried thyme, rosemary, or tarragon, optional

¼ to ½ cup (60 ml to 120 ml) water

Process the garlic, red wine vinegar, balsamic vinegar, sugar, salt, pepper, and thyme, if using, in a blender until smooth. Add the water, 1 tablespoon at a time, to thin to the desired consistency. (You'll likely need about ¼ cup/60 ml.) Refrigerate in an airtight container for up to 5 days.

Tip: Roast a head of garlic when you already have the oven on (375 to 400°F/190 to 200°C) for another dish. Slice the top off the head of garlic, wrap tightly in parchment paper, and bake for 30 to 45 minutes. (For soft, sweet garlic with little to no browning, roast it for 30 minutes. For a deeper, darker flavor, roast for the full 45 minutes.) Let it cool slightly, then squeeze the garlic into a small bowl. Refrigerate for up to 5 days.

OFO XS GF FF

LEMON-THYME DRESSING

SERVES: 4 to 6 / Makes about ⅔ cup (180 ml) // **TIME:** 5 minutes

This is one of the few dressings in the book that calls for the traditional amount of oil in a vinaigrette. However, plain hummus and a touch of tahini yield a creamy alternative, so that's the oil-free option here.

Combine the lemon juice, thyme, garlic, sesame oil, sugar, salt, and pepper in a jar with a tight-fitting lid. (OF: Add the tahini as well.) Whisk in the oil in a slow, steady stream and adjust the seasoning. Refrigerate for up to 5 days. (Remove the garlic clove before serving.)

NOTE: *Use a halved garlic clove in place of minced when you want just a hint of garlic flavor in a dressing, as we did here. Remove the garlic before serving.*

⅓ cup (80 ml) fresh lemon juice (about 2 lemons)

2 sprigs fresh thyme, leaves stripped and chopped, stems discarded

1 garlic clove, sliced in half (see Note)

1 teaspoon sesame oil (OF: 1 teaspoon GF tahini)

½ teaspoon sugar

½ teaspoon salt

Pinch black pepper

¼ cup (60 ml) olive oil (OF: ¼ cup/60 g plain GF hummus)

LIME-CUMIN DRESSING

SERVES: 2 to 4 / Makes about ½ cup (120 ml) // **TIME:** 5 minutes

Dressings are an easy way to learn how to balance seasonings (see below for more on that). This one has smoky cumin, plus sweet, sour, acidic, and salty flavors. You can use this dressing not only on a taco salad but also as a marinade for tempeh and root vegetables. Or drizzle it on cooked grains or a Lifesaving Bowl (page 88). Add cilantro or basil for a new flavor.

1 teaspoon ground cumin

1 teaspoon sugar

¼ teaspoon salt

3 tablespoons fresh lime juice
    (from 2 limes)

1 tablespoon apple cider vinegar

¼ cup (60 ml) extra virgin olive oil
    (OF: ½ avocado, pureed)

Combine the cumin, sugar, and salt in a medium jar with a tight-fitting lid. Whisk in the lime juice and vinegar. (OF: Add the avocado as well.) Whisk in the oil in a slow, steady stream. Refrigerate for up to 4 days. (Use the avocado version within 1 day.) Shake to combine as needed.

> **Tip:** There are five basic flavors: sweet, salty, sour, bitter, and umami. Dishes that we consider "delicious" are those that provide a balanced contrast between these flavors. Salad dressings, especially vinaigrettes, are a great way to practice your seasoning skills. Taste as you go along, and trust your taste buds. Is something too salty or sour? Add more sweetness. Too bland? Add acid, which lends a sour flavor. Is it missing some oomph? You're likely in need of umami. As you "take off the training wheels" and start cooking without a recipe, this skill will mean the difference between ho-hum meals and "Oh, wow!" ones.

CREAMY AVOCADO-LIME DRESSING

SERVES: 4 to 6 / Makes about 2 cups (480 ml) // **TIME:** 5 minutes

Thanks to the avocado, this dressing is creamy and rich without any added oil. There's quite a bit of tang from the lime juice, so it pairs well with heavier fare like Mexican food. It also can be used as the dressing in a massaged kale salad.

Process all the ingredients in a high-speed blender until smooth. Adjust the seasoning and add the water, 1 tablespoon at a time, plus more as needed to achieve the desired consistency (up to an additional ¼ cup/60 ml). Use within 1 day.

1 avocado, diced

¼ cup (60 ml) fresh lime or lemon juice (about 2 limes or lemons)

¼ cup (4 g) cilantro leaves

½ teaspoon ground cumin

¼ teaspoon salt

½ cup (120 ml) water, plus more as needed

YOU WON'T BELIEVE IT'S CASHEW RANCH DRESSING

SERVES: 8 to 12 / Makes about 2½ cups (600 ml) // **TIME:** 5 minutes, not including time to soak cashews

Certified nutritionist Sid Garza-Hillman, author of *Approaching the Natural*, bills himself as "The Small-Step Advocate," advising an approach to habit change that's right in line with ours. Matt and his wife, Erin, credit this creamy dressing of Sid's with making salad lovers of their kids, just as it has with many of Sid's clients. Even hard-core ranch dressing fans have a hard time believing this one is vegan, not to mention (mostly) raw! We are thrilled Sid is letting us share it with you. For a creamier dressing, soak the cashews for 1 to 2 hours before using.

1¼ cups (150 g) raw cashews (soaked for 1 to 2 hours, if desired)

¾ cup (180 ml) water, plus more as needed

1 tablespoon plus 1½ teaspoons fresh lemon juice

1 tablespoon apple cider vinegar

1½ teaspoons onion powder

1 teaspoon dried dill

1 teaspoon salt

½ teaspoon dried basil

½ teaspoon garlic powder

¼ teaspoon black pepper

Process all the ingredients in a high-speed blender until smooth. Adjust the seasoning if necessary, and add additional water, 1 tablespoon at a time, as needed to achieve the desired consistency (up to ¼ cup/60 ml). Refrigerate in an airtight container up for up to 1 week. (The dressing will thicken in the refrigerator; stir in water as needed to thin before serving.)

CLASSIC FRENCH VINAIGRETTE

SERVES: 2 to 4 / Makes about ½ cup (120 ml) // **TIME:** 5 minutes

This authentic dressing was passed down by the woman who hosted Stepf when she lived in the Loire Valley. It's been modified over the years, with balsamic and thyme standing in for whatever magic Madame Vavasseur sprinkled into hers. It pairs well with root vegetables and kale, as well as tender spring lettuce. It is rather heavy, so a little goes a long way.

Combine the apple cider vinegar, shallot, and balsamic vinegar in a medium jar with a tight-fitting lid. Let sit for 5 minutes. Stir in the mustard and thyme. Whisk in the oil in a slow, steady stream and season with salt and pepper to taste. Refrigerate for up to 5 days.

3 tablespoons apple cider vinegar

2 tablespoons minced shallot (or 1 tablespoon minced red onion)

1 tablespoon balsamic vinegar

1 teaspoon GF Dijon mustard

½ teaspoon dried thyme

¼ cup (60 ml) olive oil (OF: 2 tablespoons white beans pureed with 2 tablespoons water)

Salt and black pepper

MAPLE-DIJON DRESSING

SERVES: 2 to 4 / Makes about ½ cup (120 ml) // **TIME:** 5 minutes

This dressing is a staple in fall and winter. Try it with a lentil and root veggie bowl, on potato salad, or over roasted beets. If you're just not that into Dijon, scale it back and ramp up the maple. If you want to add herbs, rosemary and thyme are good choices.

¼ cup (60 ml) apple cider vinegar

2 tablespoons maple syrup

2 teaspoons GF Dijon mustard

¼ teaspoon black pepper

2 tablespoons olive oil
(OF: 2 tablespoons broth
or water)

Salt

Combine the vinegar, maple syrup, mustard, and pepper (OF: add the broth at this point) in a small jar with a tight-fitting lid. Whisk in the oil in a slow, steady stream. Season with salt to taste. Refrigerate for up to 5 days.

BLUEBERRY-WALNUT VINAIGRETTE

SERVES: 2 to 4 / Makes about 1 cup (240 ml) // **TIME:** 5 minutes

Fruit dressings can be cloyingly sweet, but this oil-free version embraces the natural bitterness of walnuts to balance the sweet tang of the blueberries. It's slightly chunky and complements bitter greens well; try it on arugula or atop roasted root vegetables. Pair this dressing with some crumbled soft nut-based vegan cheese on any salad.

1 Puree the vinegar, blueberries, and half of the walnuts in a blender until smooth, thinning it with 1 or 2 tablespoons of water if desired.

2 Finely chop the rest of the walnuts. Transfer to a jar with a tight-fitting lid and add the shallot, thyme, and sugar. Shake to combine and season with salt and pepper. Refrigerate for at least a few hours and up to 3 days to allow the flavors to meld.

¼ cup (60 ml) apple cider vinegar

¼ cup (40 g) blueberries

¼ cup (30 g) walnut pieces

1 or 2 tablespoons water, optional

1 tablespoon minced shallot or red onion

½ teaspoon dried thyme

½ teaspoon sugar or maple syrup

Salt and black pepper

CREAMY HERBED HEMP DRESSING

SERVES: 4 to 6 / Makes 1½ cups (360 ml) // **TIME:** 10 minutes

This is basically goddess dressing made with hemp seeds. If you prefer a dressing with more texture (and one that is less green in color), fold in the scallion, dill, and parsley after blending. In summer, drizzle this over fresh tomatoes and cucumbers. In winter, use it on roasted potatoes or as a dip for Baked Tempeh Nuggets (page 170).

½ cup (80 g) hemp seeds

¼ cup (15 g) chopped flat-leaf parsley

2 tablespoons raw cashews

1 scallion (white and light green part), sliced

1 tablespoon apple cider vinegar

1 tablespoon fresh lemon juice

2 teaspoons capers, drained

1 teaspoon nutritional yeast

½ teaspoon garlic powder

½ teaspoon sugar, optional

¼ teaspoon dried dill

Salt and black pepper

1 or 2 tablespoons water, optional

Process the hemp seeds, parsley, cashews, scallion, vinegar, lemon juice, capers, nutritional yeast, garlic powder, sugar, and dill in a high-speed blender until smooth. Season with salt and pepper and add water, 1 tablespoon at a time, as needed to achieve desired consistency. Refrigerate in an airtight container for up to 5 days.

Chapter 6

SMALL PLATES & SIDES

Most people who go vegan notice an unexpected phenomenon: Your meals become one-dish wonders. Whereas it used to be a meat, a starch, and a vegetable, now it's often just a big bowl of plant-based goodness—which could be a hearty pasta dish, a tofu-and-veggie stir-fry, a giant salad with quinoa and beans, or one of infinite combinations of "a grain, a green, and a bean."

The point is, it's really easy to go down this one-dish road. Nutrition takes center stage. Cooking and cleanup are simple. And hey, who wants to plan and shop for three dishes when you can get the job done with one? But even if every bite remains delicious when you eat this way, there's no denying that every bite is, well, the same.

We don't mean to knock this simple approach to food. Simplifying mealtime has been one of the joys of our plant-based journeys, and the minimalist mind-set has even spilled over into other areas of our lives. But that doesn't mean a plant-based diet can't be every bit as interesting and entertaining as other ways of eating when we want it to be.

The side dishes in this section are meant to add variety to your diet—not so much for nutrition's sake, but for fun (and your sanity). Use the recipes here to round out a meal, or create an entire tapas-style feast with whole grain and veggie side dishes. These small plates are designed to be quick and flavorful; they're a simple way to make your weekday meals more varied and memorable without a lot of effort.

And if you decide to stick to your simple ways and just make a giant portion of Tahini Green Beans (page 158), Potato-Stuffed Portobellos (page 169), or Olive-Chickpea Waffles (page 178) and call it yet another one-dish dinner, well, we can't say we haven't done the same.

TAHINI GREEN BEANS

SERVES: 2 to 4 // **TIME:** 15 minutes

This recipe quickly entered regular rotation for everyone who tested it; the tahini and sesame seeds make green beans incredibly enticing with very little effort. If you are a dipper, serve the sauce on the side and eat the green beans like fries. This technique also works with steamed or roasted broccoli, cauliflower, carrots, or beets.

1 pound (454 g) green beans, washed and trimmed

2 tablespoons GF tahini

1 garlic clove, minced

Grated zest and juice of 1 lemon

Salt and black pepper

1 teaspoon toasted black or white sesame seeds, optional

1 Steam the beans in a medium saucepan fitted with a steamer insert (or by adding ¼ cup/60 ml water to a covered saucepan) over medium-high heat. Drain, reserving the cooking water.

2 Mix the tahini, garlic, lemon zest and juice, and salt and pepper to taste. Use the reserved cooking water to thin the sauce as desired.

3 Toss the green beans with the sauce and serve warm or at room temperature. Garnish with the sesame seeds, if using.

FF: *Use a pound of frozen French-style haricots verts. Run them under hot water until thawed, and drain well.*

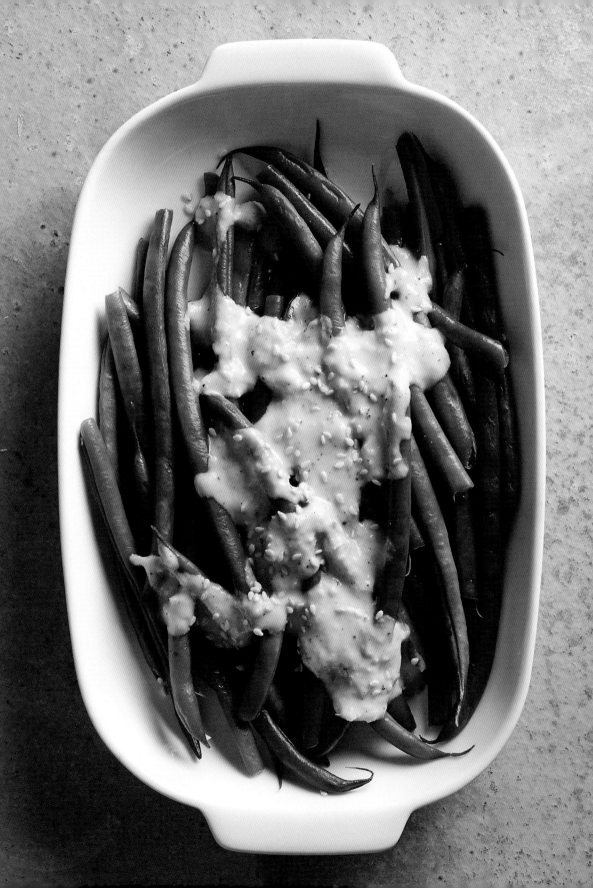

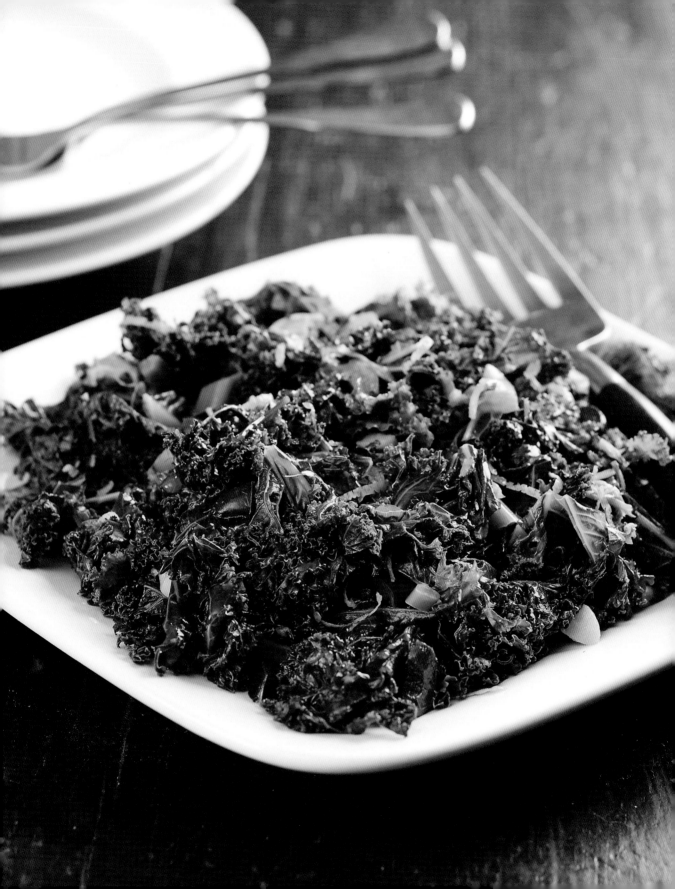

LEMONY STEAMED KALE WITH OLIVES

SERVES: 2 to 4 // **TIME:** 10 minutes to prep, 20 minutes to cook

This dish is based on Spanish herb "jam," which is traditionally loaded with olive oil. In our lighter version, we add plenty of fresh herbs to steamed greens and layer on flavor with the combo of lemon and olives. If you use the celery leaves, this dish takes advantage of what would otherwise be compost or trash. Serve on toast with plain hummus.

1 Place the kale, celery leaves, parsley, and garlic in a steamer basket set over a medium saucepan. Steam over medium-high heat, covered, for 15 minutes. Remove from the heat and squeeze out any excess moisture.

2 Place a large skillet over medium heat. Add the oil, then add the kale mixture to the skillet. Cook, stirring often, for 5 minutes.

3 Remove from the heat and add the olives and lemon zest and juice. Season with salt and pepper and serve. (This dish can be served warm, cold, or at room temperature.)

1 bunch kale, leaves chopped and stems minced

½ cup (30 g) celery leaves, roughly chopped, or additional parsley

½ bunch flat-leaf parsley, stems and leaves roughly chopped

4 garlic cloves, chopped

2 teaspoons olive oil (OF: 2 tablespoons broth)

¼ cup (45 g) pitted Kalamata olives, chopped

Grated zest and juice of 1 lemon

Salt and pepper

ZUCCHINI "PARMESAN"

SERVES: 2 to 4 // **TIME:** 10 minutes to prep, 20 minutes to bake

Zucchini Parmesan with homemade marinara is a summer classic. This version is less labor-intensive, with no oil (or actual Parmesan, of course). Any leftovers could become a layer in lasagna! Serve this dish with Weeknight Marinara (page 81) if desired.

4 zucchini, sliced into ½-inch (13 mm) rounds

½ cup (120 ml) almond milk

1 teaspoon arrowroot powder

1 teaspoon fresh lemon juice

½ teaspoon salt

½ cup (55 g) whole wheat bread crumbs (see Note)

¼ cup (40 g) hemp seeds

¼ cup (15 g) nutritional yeast

½ teaspoon garlic powder

¼ teaspoon black pepper

¼ teaspoon crushed red pepper

1 Preheat the oven to 375°F (190°C). Line two baking sheets with parchment paper.

2 Place the zucchini in a medium bowl with the almond milk, arrowroot powder, lemon juice, and ¼ teaspoon of the salt. Stir to combine.

3 Combine the bread crumbs, hemp seeds, nutritional yeast, garlic powder, black pepper, and crushed red pepper in a large bowl with a lid. Add the zucchini in batches and shake until the slices are evenly coated.

4 Place the zucchini in a single layer on the prepared baking sheets. Bake until the zucchini slices are golden brown, about 20 minutes. Serve.

NOTE: *Use panko (Japanese bread crumbs) for more crunch.*

CASHEW CREAMED KALE

SERVES: 2 to 4 // **TIME:** 5 minutes to prep, 10 minutes to cook, not including time to make Cashew Cream

A little bit of fat helps your body absorb the goodness from greens, and the richness of the Cashew Cream takes the flavor of simple steamed vegetables up a notch. This is more of a blueprint than a recipe; instead of kale, try broccoli, cauliflower, or any cruciferous vegetables you have on hand.

Add the kale, lemon juice, and garlic to a medium skillet set over medium heat and season with salt and pepper. Add the water. Cook, covered, for 5 minutes, then start checking for desired doneness. When the kale is tender enough for your liking, stir in the cashew cream until thoroughly coated. Serve.

1 bunch kale, stemmed and chopped

1 teaspoon fresh lemon juice

1 clove garlic, minced

Pinch of salt

Black pepper

2 tablespoons water

2 tablespoons Cashew Cream (page 236)

COLCANNON

SERVES: 4 to 6 // **TIME:** 20 minutes, not including time to make Cashew Cream

Yeah, we know the real-deal Irish dish doesn't have lemon or nutmeg in it. But those ingredients, plus Cashew Cream, elevate humble cabbage and potatoes to a level that's worth raising a pint of (soon-to-be-vegan!) Guinness to.

6 waxy potatoes,
  such as Yukon Gold

¼ head cabbage, red or green,
  roughly chopped

¼ teaspoon freshly grated nutmeg

Grated zest from 1 lemon

¼ cup (40 g) Cashew Cream
  (page 236)

Salt and black pepper

1 Steam or boil the potatoes in a large pot with a lid over medium-high heat until fork-tender, about 15 minutes.

2 While the potatoes cook, steam the cabbage in a medium saucepan with a lid over medium-high heat until tender, about 10 minutes. (You can do this on top of the potatoes if you have a steamer with multiple baskets.)

3 Drain the potatoes and mash. Fold in the cabbage, nutmeg, lemon zest, and cashew cream. Season with salt and pepper and serve.

Variation: For Kale-cannon, use 2 bunches kale in place of the cabbage.

BLUEPRINT: PAKORAS

MAKES: 24 pakoras // **TIME:** 15 minutes to prep, 30 minutes to bake

Those deep-fried veggie fritters you can find at most any Indian restaurant are so good, but they're also loaded with oil and salt. These baked ones are heavy on the veggies and use no oil! Pair them with Cashew Tzatziki (page 239), chili garlic sauce, or a jarred chutney.

① Preheat the oven to 425°F (220°C). Line two baking sheets with parchment paper.

② Combine the flour, garam masala, baking powder, turmeric, and ½ teaspoon salt in a large bowl, then whisk in the water. Fold in the vegetables.

③ Scoop golf ball-size portions onto the prepared baking sheets. Bake until the pakoras are golden brown and the edges are crispy, about 25 minutes, rotating the baking sheets half-way through. Sprinkle with additional salt if desired and serve. (Leftovers can be refrigerated for up to 3 days and reheated in a 300°F/150°C oven.)

NOTE: *You might notice we also have a recipe for Samosa Burgers (see page 105), another Indian appetizer that usually involves deep-frying. Samosas are traditionally spiced mashed potatoes and peas wrapped in a wheat dough, while pakoras are a chickpea flour batter with veggies mixed in.*

2 cups (240 g) chickpea flour
   (garbanzo bean flour)

2 tablespoons Garam Masala
   (page 223)

1 teaspoon GF baking powder

1 teaspoon ground turmeric

½ teaspoon salt, plus more
   to taste, optional

1½ cups (360 ml) water

5 to 6 cups (445 to 535 g) mixed
   vegetables (choose as few or as
   many as you'd like)

» thinly sliced cabbage

» quartered button or cremini
   mushrooms

» finely chopped yellow onion

» shredded beets or carrots

» chopped broccoli or
   cauliflower

» diced bell pepper

» chopped kale, spinach,
   or mixed greens

CUMIN-CITRUS ROASTED CARROTS

SERVES: 4 to 6 // **TIME:** 10 minutes to prep, 30 minutes to bake

Carrots have a lot of natural sweetness, and roasting them really highlights this quality. Here, we add a combo of lime and orange juice plus smoky cumin for an oil-free sauce with no need for added sugar.

8 large carrots, sliced into ½-inch (13 mm) rounds

¼ cup (60 ml) orange juice

¼ cup (60 ml) vegetable broth

1 teaspoon ground cumin

¼ teaspoon ground turmeric

Salt and black pepper

1 tablespoon fresh lime juice

Chopped flat-leaf parsley, optional

1 Preheat the oven to 400°F (200°C).

2 Place the carrots in a large baking dish, then add the orange juice, broth, cumin, and turmeric. Season with salt and pepper.

3 Bake, uncovered, until the carrots are lightly browned and the juices have reduced slightly, about 30 minutes, stirring halfway through. Drizzle with the lime juice and parsley, if using, and serve.

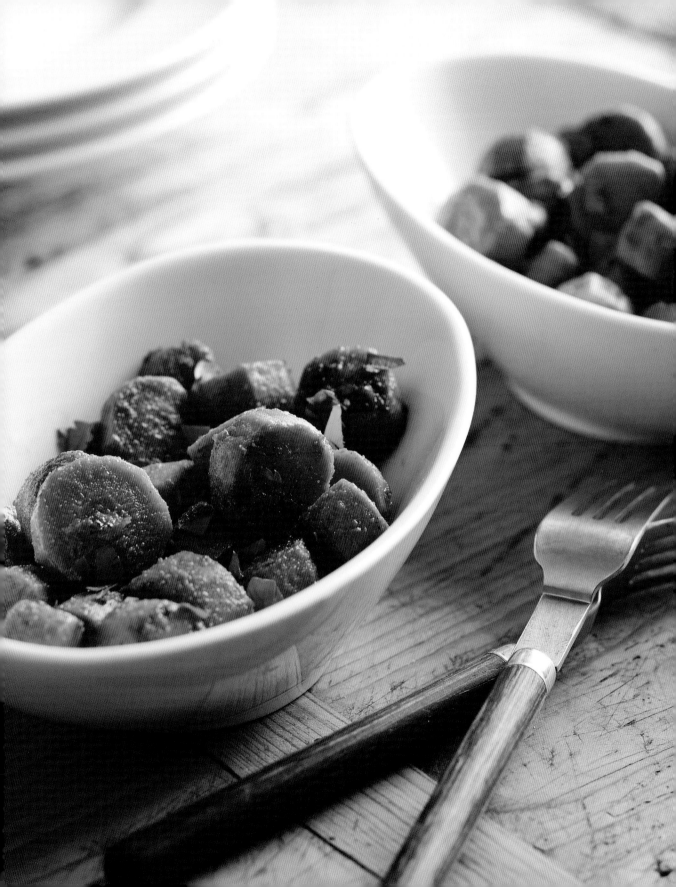

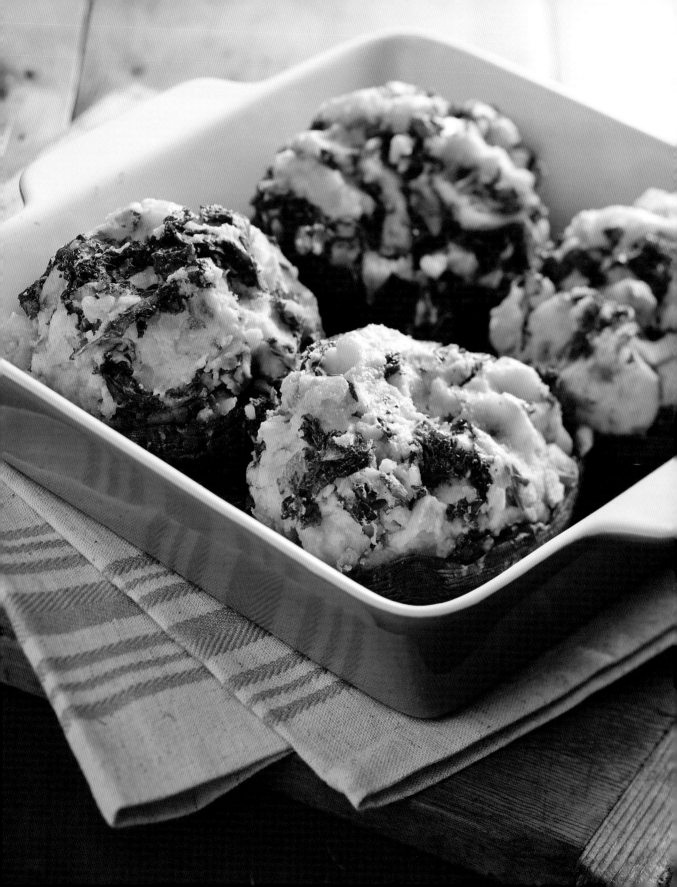

POTATO-STUFFED PORTOBELLOS

MAKES: 4 stuffed mushrooms // **TIME:** 45 minutes,
not including time to marinate or make B-Savory Sauce and Kale-cannon

This is such a simple dish, but it does require some planning so the 'shrooms can soak up all the marinade. It feels slightly upscale without being fussy and requires almost no hands-on work, making it a perfect dinner party option.

1 Place the mushrooms in a shallow dish, stemmed side up. Pour the marinade on top and turn them as needed to thoroughly coat. Cover and refrigerate for at least 8 hours or overnight.

2 Preheat the oven to 400°F (200°C). Transfer the portobellos to a medium baking dish and carefully stuff each with a quarter of the kale-cannon.

3 Bake, covered, for 15 minutes. While the mushrooms bake, combine the water and arrowroot powder. Remove the mushrooms from the oven and add the arrowroot mixture to the bottom of the baking dish. Use a spatula to scrape down the sides. Continue to bake until the mushrooms are soft and the potatoes are heated through, about 20 minutes. Serve.

4 large portobello mushroom caps, stems removed

¼ cup (60 ml) B-Savory Sauce & Marinade (page 232)

1 batch Kale-cannon (page 164)

½ cup (120 ml) water or vegetable broth

1 teaspoon arrowroot powder

BAKED TEMPEH NUGGETS

SERVES: 2 to 4 // **TIME:** 15 minutes to prepare, 30 minutes to bake

These are crunchy, chewy little nuggets that even picky kids will gobble up. Lightly steaming the tempeh reduces its bitterness. Use soy-free tempeh (Yes, it's a thing! We like Smiling Hara Black-Eyed Pea Tempeh.) and/or gluten-free bread crumbs if necessary. Wrap leftovers in a whole-grain tortilla with sprouts, shredded carrots, and a drizzle of Creamy Herbed Hemp Dressing (page 156) for a quick lunch.

One 8-ounce (227 g) package tempeh, lightly steamed if desired

¼ cup (60 ml) almond milk

¼ cup (15 g) nutritional yeast

1 tablespoon Fall & Winter All-Purpose Seasoning (page 229) or other seasoning blend

1 teaspoon arrowroot powder

1 teaspoon fresh lemon juice

¼ teaspoon black pepper

¼ teaspoon hot sauce

¼ teaspoon salt

1 cup (110 g) whole wheat bread crumbs (see Note)

1 Preheat the oven to 400°F (200°C). Line a baking sheet with parchment paper.

2 Slice the tempeh in half and then quarter each half to form 8 pieces. Smash each one slightly with the heel of your hand to increase surface area and make them more nugget-like.

3 In a shallow dish, combine the almond milk, nutritional yeast, seasoning blend, arrowroot powder, lemon juice, pepper, hot sauce, and salt. Add the tempeh nuggets and allow to soak for 5 minutes, turning them to get each piece well coated.

4 Place the bread crumbs in another shallow dish. Using one hand for the wet and one for the dry, transfer each piece of tempeh from the batter to the bread crumbs. Place on the prepared baking sheet.

5 Bake for 30 minutes, flipping halfway, until golden brown on both sides. Serve.

NOTE: *For more crunch, use panko (Japanese bread crumbs).*

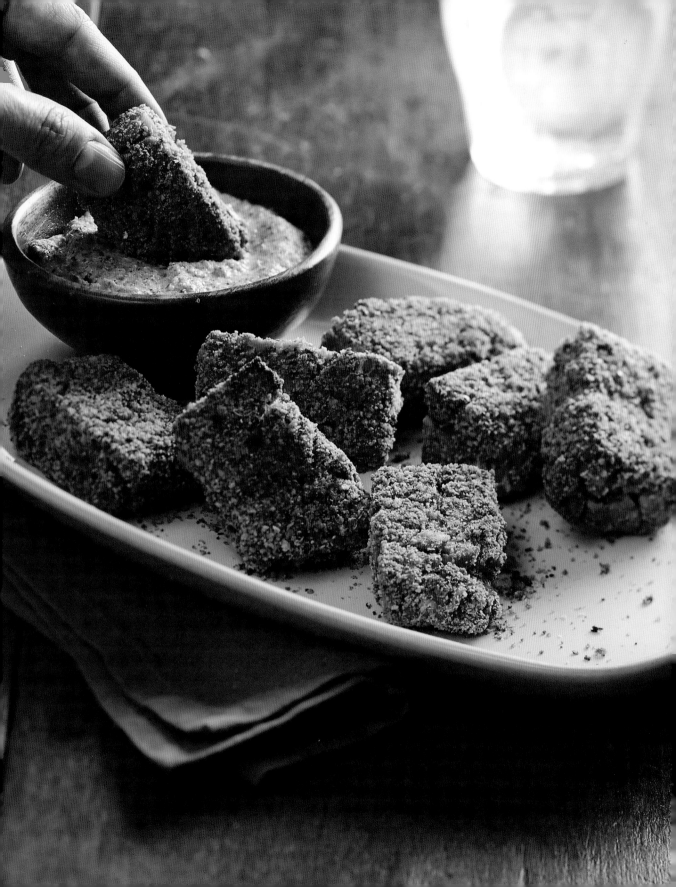

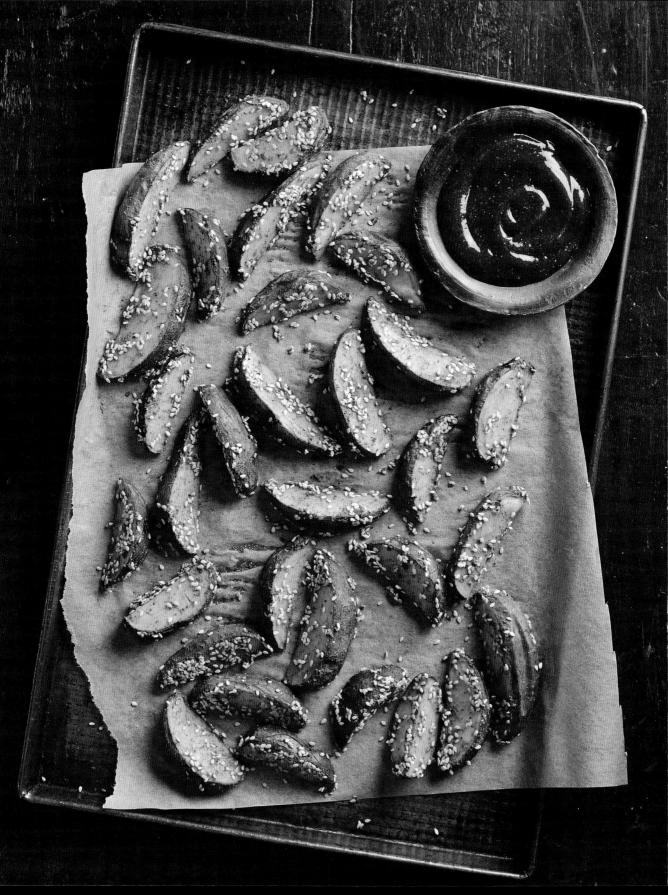

SESAME-TURMERIC OVEN FRIES

SERVES: 2 to 4 // **TIME:** 10 minutes to prep, 30 minutes to bake

These are a match made in heaven with Spicy Black Bean & Beet Burgers (page 108). They become crisp with very little oil (and can be made without any oil at all), and they are coated with a seasoning blend that borders on addictive. The trick is the arrowroot powder, which binds with the starch in the potatoes and helps the seasonings adhere while ensuring crispy baked "fries." We like to serve these fries with Curry Ketchup (see Tip) or Miso Gravy (page 231).

1 Preheat the oven to 375°F (190°C). Line a baking sheet with parchment paper.

2 Combine the arrowroot powder, turmeric, cumin, garlic powder, salt, and pepper in a medium bowl. Add the potatoes and toss well to combine, until all cut surfaces are coated with the spice mixture. (They should start to turn yellow from the turmeric.) Let sit while the oven preheats.

3 Toss the potatoes once more, then pour off any excess moisture that may have accumulated in the bottom of the bowl. (This will help the potatoes crisp.) Add the oil and sesame seeds and toss the potatoes to coat.

4 Pour the potatoes onto the prepared baking sheet in a single layer. Scrape the bowl to get all the sesame seeds onto the potatoes. Bake for 30 minutes, or until crispy and golden brown. Serve.

1 teaspoon arrowroot powder

1 teaspoon ground turmeric

¾ teaspoon ground cumin

½ teaspoon garlic powder

½ teaspoon salt

¼ teaspoon black pepper

5 to 6 red potatoes (about 1 pound/455 g), cut into wedges or bite-size pieces

1 tablespoon grapeseed or melted coconut oil (OF: 1 tablespoon broth)

2 tablespoons sesame seeds

> **Tip:** This two-ingredient Curry Ketchup is a simple, memorable sauce. Mix 1 teaspoon yellow curry powder into ¼ cup (60 g) ketchup (no sugar added, reduced-sodium preferred).

SLOW-COOKER REFRIED BEANS

SERVES: 6 to 8 // **TIME:** 5 minutes to prep, 4 to 8 hours to cook, not including time to soak beans

Beans are nutritional powerhouses worth building into your daily diet, and "refried" beans are a delicious and satisfying way to help to make that happen. Using the slow cooker means prep is next to nil—you can even let these cook overnight! Onion and smoky cumin pack these beans with flavor, and oregano stands in for epazote, a traditional herb that can be hard to find. Kombu adds depth of flavor and increases digestibility of legumes as they cook.

1 pound (454 g) pinto or black beans, soaked all day or overnight, drained, and rinsed

1 yellow onion, minced or grated

3 garlic cloves, minced

1-inch (2.5 cm) strip kombu

1 tablespoon olive oil (OF: omit)

1 tablespoon plus 1 teaspoon ground cumin

½ teaspoon dried oregano

½ teaspoon smoked paprika

6 to 8 (1.4 to 2 L) cups water

½ teaspoon salt, or to taste

1 Add the beans, onion, garlic, kombu, oil, cumin, oregano, and paprika to a slow cooker, along with the water. (Use more water if your slow cooker is hot—see Tip—or if you're letting them cook overnight or while you're away from home.) Turn on high for 8 hours or overnight.

2 If necessary, drain and reserve the water (this won't affect the flavor), then mash with a potato masher or puree in a food processor. (If the beans are too thick, add the reserved cooking water a tablespoon at a time. If they're too thin, return to the slow cooker and cook on high for 30 minutes with the lid off to allow water to evaporate.) Season with the salt.

3 Serve or allow to cool and pack into half-pint (250 ml) jars, leaving at least ½ inch (13 mm) of space to allow for expansion, and freeze for up to 3 months.

Variation: For spicy beans, add 1 to 2 GF chipotle chiles in adobo sauce, chopped, or 1 minced jalapeño.

> **Tip:** Every brand and every size of slow cooker will heat things a little differently. To allow for this, we give a time range for our slow-cooker recipes. For example, the popular Instant Pot's slow-cooker setting is quite hot and cooks things faster than a traditional cooker does. For best results, err on the side of shorter cooking time but allow for the max, and use the upper end of the water recommendation if your slow cooker tends to run hot.

UGLY VEGGIE MASH

SERVES: 6 to 8 // **TIME:** 10 minutes to prep, 25 minutes to cook

Beauty is only skin-deep when it comes to root veggies. This dish honors three of the most under-appreciated—and least attractive—roots in the produce department. Celeriac (celery root) is creamy with a delicate celery taste. Rutabagas have a texture akin to a waxy potato with a slight spice, similar to a turnip. (They need to be peeled because their purple-and-white skin is often waxed to lengthen shelf life.) And parsnips are pale, sweeter cousins of the carrot. Simmered in broth and roughly mashed together, this motley crew becomes a delightful alternative to mashed potatoes. You can substitute other root vegetables as desired, even adding white potatoes. For a richer dish, stir in ¼ cup (40 g) Cashew Cream (page 236).

1 Place the parsnips, rutabaga, and celeriac in a large pot with a tight-fitting lid. Add the broth, cover, and bring to a boil over high heat. Reduce the heat to low and cook until the vegetables are fork-tender and most of the liquid has evaporated, 20 to 25 minutes.

2 Mash with a potato masher or serving fork, season with salt and pepper, and serve.

1 pound (455 g) parsnips, peeled, trimmed, and cut into 1-inch (2.5 cm) pieces

1 large rutabaga, peeled and chopped into 1-inch (2.5 cm) cubes

1 large celeriac (celery root), peeled using a paring knife and chopped into 1-inch (2.5 cm) cubes

2 cups (480 ml) vegetable broth, such as Better than Bone Broth (page 210)

Salt and black pepper

ORZO "RISOTTO"

SERVES: 4 to 6 // **TIME:** 25 minutes

Tiny pasta such as orzo takes about half the time to cook as Arborio rice—the traditional choice for risotto—but the cooking method yields an equally creamy outcome. This side dish goes well with Nut-Crusted Tofu (page 111) or a sprinkle of pistachios. It's ready in less than 30 minutes, so you can enjoy carb-loading without spending all night in the kitchen.

4 cups (960 ml) vegetable broth

1 tablespoon olive oil (OF: omit)

1 large shallot or ¼ yellow onion, minced

1 teaspoon dried tarragon or dill

1 pound (455 g) whole wheat orzo

½ cup (120 ml) white wine, or 1 tablespoon apple cider vinegar plus ⅓ cup (80 ml) vegetable broth

Grated zest and juice of 1 lemon

Salt and black pepper

Chopped flat-leaf parsley, optional

1 Bring the broth to a boil in a medium saucepan; reduce the heat to medium-low and cover.

2 Place a large saucepan over medium heat. Add the oil to the pan, then add the shallot. Cover and cook, stirring often, until the shallot is soft and translucent, about 5 minutes. Stir in the tarragon, followed by the orzo.

3 Add the wine and stir the orzo constantly until the wine is absorbed.

4 Continuing to stir constantly, add the broth 1 cup (240 ml) at a time. The orzo will absorb the broth, which should take about 3 to 5 minutes, and begin to get creamy. Repeat with the remaining broth.

5 Remove from the heat, stir in the lemon zest and juice, and season with salt and pepper. Garnish with the parsley, if using, and serve.

BAKED BROWN RICE RISOTTO WITH SUNFLOWER SEEDS

SERVES: 4 to 6 // **TIME:** 10 minutes to prep, 1 hour to bake

Risotto is unbelievably satisfying, but who has an hour to spend at the stove trying to coax a pot of rice into creamy submission? This baked variety is almost as creamy but requires a fraction of the work. Sunflower seeds provide a nutrient boost and textural contrast.

1 Preheat the oven to 400°F (200°C). Bring the broth to a boil in a medium saucepan.

2 Add the rice, sunflower seeds, sherry, shallot, tarragon, dill, salt, pepper, and turmeric to a medium baking dish. Pour the hot broth into the dish, cover, and carefully place in the oven. Bake for 30 minutes. The dish should still look soupy; if it begins to dry out, add 1 cup (240 ml) of water or broth. Continue to bake, covered, for another 30 minutes. Serve.

Variation: For Pumpkin-Sage Risotto, substitute 1 tablespoon dried sage for the dill and tarragon, then stir in 1 cup (245 g) pumpkin puree halfway through the cooking process.

4 cups (960 ml) vegetable broth

1 cup (180 g) short-grain brown rice

½ cup (75 g) raw sunflower seeds

2 tablespoons dry sherry or ¼ cup (60 ml) white wine

1 shallot, minced

1 teaspoon dried tarragon

½ teaspoon dried dill

½ teaspoon salt (use half this if your broth is salted)

⅛ teaspoon black pepper

⅛ teaspoon ground turmeric

OLIVE-CHICKPEA WAFFLES

MAKES: 4 to 6 waffles // **TIME:** 10 minutes to prep, 30 minutes to cook

Soccas are Mediterranean flatbreads made with chickpea flour. But although they are quick to make and full of nutrition from the chickpeas, they typically call for quite a bit of olive oil to add flavor and richness. Inspired by socca but seeking something lighter, we created these savory waffles.

2 cups (240 g) chickpea flour (garbanzo bean flour)

1 tablespoon chopped rosemary or thyme

1 teaspoon GF baking powder

¼ teaspoon salt

⅛ teaspoon black pepper

½ cup (90 g) pitted Kalamata olives, chopped

¼ cup (15 g) sun-dried tomatoes, thinly sliced

1 tablespoon olive oil (OF: omit)

1½ cups (360 ml) hot water

Hummus or Weeknight Marinara (page 81)

1 Preheat a waffle iron. (OF: See page 49 for baking directions if your waffle iron isn't truly nonstick.)

2 Combine the flour, rosemary, baking powder, salt, and pepper in a large bowl. Stir in the olives and sun-dried tomatoes, then whisk in the oil followed by the hot water. The batter should be thick but thoroughly combined.

3 Spread about ½ to ¾ cup (120 to 180 ml) batter onto the waffle iron, close the lid, and cook through, according to waffle iron directions, about 6 minutes.

4 Top with hummus and serve.

Variation: Substitute ½ cup (30 g) chopped flat-leaf parsley for the olives and fold in ¼ cup (40 g) chopped red onion.

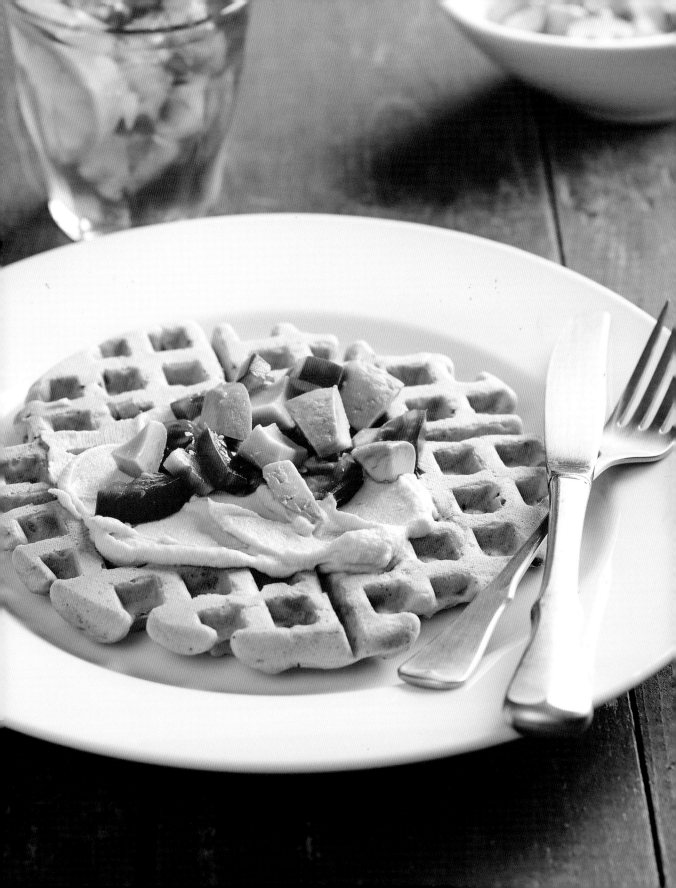

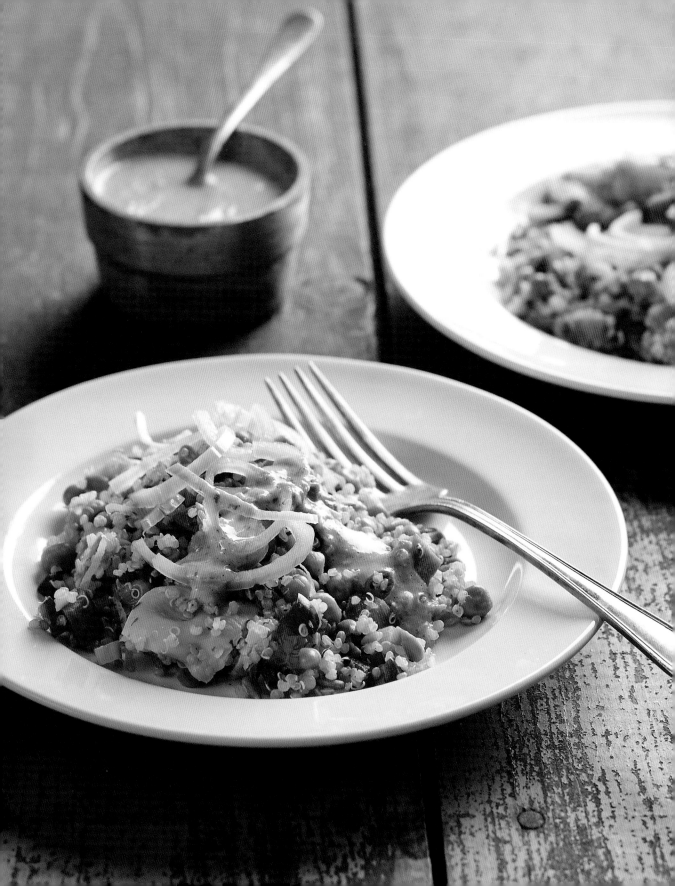

OF XS GF FF

QUINOA PRIMAVERA

SERVES: 4 to 6 // **TIME:** 25 minutes

Quinoa is the rare plant protein that contains all nine essential amino acids, making it "complete." Whether this actually matters is up for debate, but quinoa certainly rounds out a lot of our meals. Paired with loads of vegetables, this dish becomes a one-pot meal. If you need a sauce, try it with the Green on Greens Dressing (page 145).

1 **To make the shallots,** combine all the ingredients in a small bowl. Refrigerate until ready to serve. (The shallots can be refrigerated overnight or up to 3 days.)

2 **To make the quinoa,** combine the water and quinoa in a large saucepan over high heat. Bring to a boil, then add the artichokes, garlic, tarragon, thyme, ½ teaspoon salt, the dill, and ¼ teaspoon pepper. Reduce the heat to medium-low, cover, and cook for 10 minutes. Reduce the heat to low and stir in the peas, carrots, bell pepper, and scallions. Cover and cook until the vegetables are heated through, about 5 minutes.

3 Remove from the heat, add the lemon juice and zest and the sunflower seeds, fluff with a fork, and season with salt and pepper. Serve, topping each portion with the shallots. (Leftovers can be served cold.)

CITRUS-PICKLED SHALLOTS

2 large shallots, sliced in half, then into half-moons
2 tablespoons orange juice
½ teaspoon apple cider vinegar
½ teaspoon salt
Pinch of sugar

QUINOA

2 cups (480 ml) water
1 cup (190 g) quinoa, soaked at least 2 hours or overnight, rinsed, and drained
2 cups (520 g) frozen artichoke hearts or one 14-ounce (400 g) can artichoke hearts packed in water, halved or quartered if large
2 garlic cloves, minced
1 teaspoon dried tarragon
½ teaspoon dried thyme
½ teaspoon salt, plus more to taste
¼ teaspoon dried dill
¼ teaspoon black pepper, plus more to taste
2 cups (250 g) frozen peas
2 carrots, diced
1 orange or yellow bell pepper, chopped fine
3 scallions (white and light green parts), sliced thin
Grated zest and juice of 1 lemon
½ cup (75 g) raw sunflower seeds

FARRO TABBOULEH

SERVES: 4 to 6 // **TIME:** 15 minutes to prep, 30 minutes to cook, not including time to soak farro

We love traditional Middle Eastern tabbouleh made with bulgur, but when we want a dish with more heft we turn to farro. Farro is an ancient grain that's readily available in most supermarkets, but you could use quinoa or pearled barley if you like. This dish gets better the longer it sits. For a full meal, toss with greens and top with beans.

2½ cups (600 ml) water or vegetable broth

1 cup (210 g) farro, soaked overnight and drained

3 scallions (white and light green parts), sliced thin

1 English cucumber, diced

1 red or yellow bell pepper, finely diced

1 bunch flat-leaf parsley, leaves only, chopped

Handful mint leaves, chopped

Grated zest and juice of 2 lemons

2 tablespoons olive oil (OF: ¼ cup/60 ml broth)

¼ teaspoon salt

⅛ teaspoon black pepper

1. Combine the water and farro in a medium saucepan. Bring to a boil, then reduce the heat to low, cover, and cook, stirring occasionally, until the farro is al dente, about 25 minutes.

2. Allow to cool for 10 minutes, then transfer to a large bowl along with the remaining ingredients. Toss to combine and serve. (The tabbouleh can be refrigerated for up to 2 days, though the herbs will discolor.).

FF: *Speed up the cool-down by spreading the cooked grains on a baking sheet. You can also use pearled farro, which will cook in just 15 minutes.*

Variation: Counting your carbs or want to amp up your veggie intake? Swap 3 cups (300 g) finely chopped raw cauliflower for the farro.

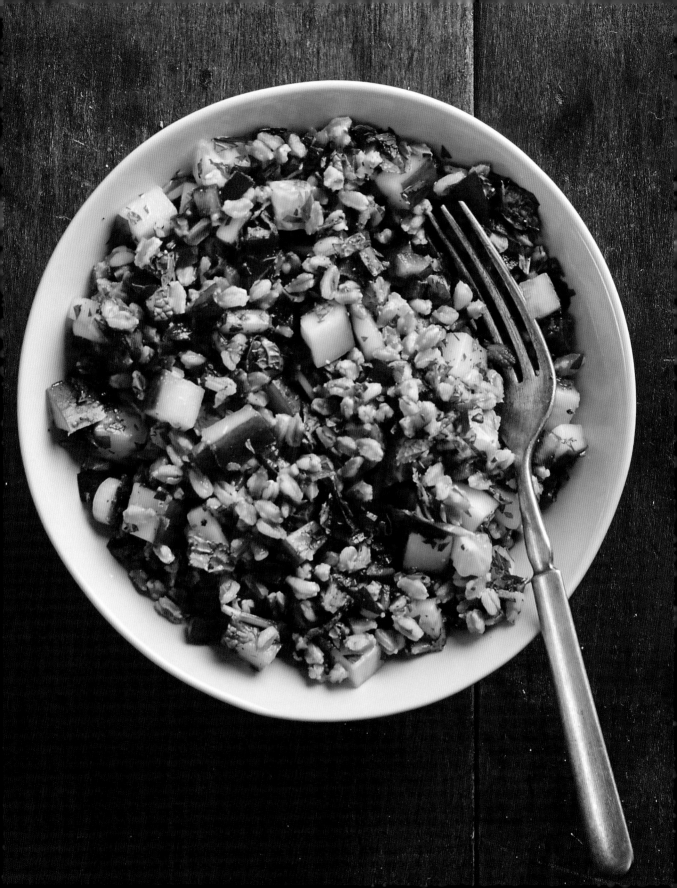

PROVENÇAL POTATO GRATIN

MAKES: 1 gratin // **TIME:** 10 minutes to prep, 40 minutes to cook

This baked potato and onion dish, based on a southern French favorite, was a sleeper hit with our recipe testers. It's delicious served warm or at room temperature and doesn't fall apart easily—making it a great choice for a mid-hike picnic.

1 tablespoon olive oil (OF: ¼ cup/60 ml broth)

2 yellow onions, thinly sliced

1 tablespoon fresh thyme, leaves only

3 garlic cloves, minced

¼ teaspoon salt, plus more to taste

2 pounds (900 g) waxy potatoes, such as Yukon Gold, sliced ¼ inch (6.5 mm) thick

One 14.5-ounce (411 g) can diced tomatoes with juice

½ cup (90 g) pitted Kalamata olives, chopped

¼ teaspoon pepper

1 Preheat the oven to 400°F (200°C).

2 Place a large skillet over medium heat. Add the oil, then add the onions and thyme and sauté until they brown slightly, about 5 minutes. Add the garlic, season with salt to taste, and remove from the heat.

3 Layer half of the onion mixture in a medium baking dish; top with the potatoes, tomatoes with their juice, and olives; then season with the ¼ teaspoon salt and ¼ teaspoon pepper. Top with the remaining onion mixture.

4 Bake, covered, for 20 minutes. Remove the lid and continue to bake until the potatoes are fully cooked and the edges start to brown, 15 to 20 minutes. Serve warm or at room temperature.

Chapter 7

FUEL & RECOVERY:
REAL FOOD FOR BEFORE, DURING & AFTER WORKOUTS

Don't undermine your workout by fueling it with processed junk that barely qualifies as food! Instead, let our recipes for natural, homemade versions of sports nutrition staples take you further so you can get the most from every workout.

TO EAT OR DRINK YOUR CARBS? THAT'S THE QUESTION

As you read in Chapter 1, you should usually only consider using added sugars and quick carbs to fuel before, during, or after a workout. For years, the only "sports drinks" on the market were loaded with refined sugar and designed to replenish carbohydrates as well as electrolytes. But for various reasons, more of today's athletes are choosing instead to eat their carbs or to forgo them altogether during workouts. As such, more lower-carb, electrolyte-only sports drinks have hit the market.

We think there's a time and a place for both types of drinks. Our new favorite sports drink, switchel—which actually isn't new at all—embraces that flexibility. Our base recipe for switchel uses just 2 tablespoons of maple syrup (100 calories, 27 g carbs), so it has about half the sugar of a traditional sports drink.

For lighter training days when you don't need an immediate energy source to get you through the workout, reach for the lower-sugar versions of switchel. On long run days, when you need more fuel, we have other switchel recipes suitable for your increased carb needs.

Our base recipe also contains 481 mg sodium from ¼ teaspoon sea salt (that's slightly lower than table salt, which has 560 mg per ¼ teaspoon), plus 129 mg potassium. It's right in line with commercial sports drinks, which typically provide 427 g sodium and 120 mg potassium in 32 ounces.

Need to customize a drink recipe? Here's a quick guide:

SODIUM:

¼ teaspoon sea salt = 481 mg sodium

1 teaspoon umeboshi (salty-sour Japanese plum paste) = 340 mg sodium

CARBOHYDRATES:

1 tablespoon maple syrup = 50 calories, 13 g carbohydrates

1 tablespoon sugar = 45 calories, 13 g carbohydrates

If you prefer another sweetener, such as dates or agave, feel free to experiment with those as well.

As you read through this chapter, you'll notice that we call some beverages "sports drinks" while others are "electrolyte drinks." The former are akin to what you'd buy at the store; the latter are designed primarily to hydrate, rather than to fuel.

Sports Drinks: Designed to be carb replacements with electrolytes

Electrolyte Drinks: Lower in carbs than traditional sports drinks

Check out this list to get started (with grams of carbs per 16 ounces):

Cucumber-Lime Electrolyte Drink: 14 g

Lemon-Lime Electrolyte Drink: 14 g

Switchel: The Original Sports Drink: 14 g

3 Switchel Mocktails: 14 g

Umeboshi Electrolyte Drink: 18 g

Miso-Maple Electrolyte "Broth": 21 g

Cranberry-Citrus Electrolyte Drink: 22 g

Fruit Punch Switchel Sports Drink with Juice: 22 g

Very Berry Switchel Sports Drink with Juice: 31 g

Orange Switchel Sports Drink with Juice: 32 g

Grape Switchel Sports Drink with Juice: 33 g

With any of these sports drinks, feel free to adjust the sweetener-to-salt ratio as needed to suit your needs and palate.

In addition, we offer recipes for solid-food fuel that contain mostly carbohydrates, or a combination of protein and carbs for extremely long workouts.

FUEL

Solid food that contains mostly carbs or a combination of carbs and protein (used during very long workouts to prevent crashes)

Calorie Bomb Cookies
(page 219)

Chocolate-Coconut-Pecan Chewy Bars
(page 220)

Green Energy Bites
(page 215)

Key Lime Pie Rice Bites
(page 217)

Piña Colada Almond Butter
(page 213)

Sesame-Tamari Portable Rice Balls
(page 214)

Strawberry Shortcake Rice Bites
(page 216)

Vegan-Edge Waffles
(page 51)

SWITCHEL: THE ORIGINAL SPORTS DRINK

GOOD FOR: hydration • before, during, and after a workout

MAKES: about 4¼ cups (1 L) // **TIME:** 5 minutes to prep, plus resting overnight

Switchel is the original sports drink, what farmers drank in the fields to stay hydrated during the summer. It's a clever combination of simple, real ingredients. Maple syrup contains magnesium and potassium, which help to prevent cramps, and the apple cider vinegar prevents nausea, stomach upset, and indigestion. (You really want raw, unfiltered apple cider vinegar here, so you get the minerals and other good stuff.) The ginger adds flavor and also helps with nausea. The drink is refreshing, mildly sweet, and tangy and, when made with fruit juices, tastes surprisingly like the convenience store sports drinks we grew up with. You'll want to refrigerate it overnight to allow the flavors to mellow and mingle. This recipe makes an entire pitcher; it'll keep for a few days in the fridge.

4 cups (960 ml) water

2 tablespoons apple cider vinegar

2 tablespoons maple syrup

1-inch (2.5 cm) piece ginger, minced

¼ teaspoon sea salt, or to taste

Shake all the ingredients together, refrigerate overnight, strain, and drink.

Nutrition info (for the entire recipe): Calories 110 Total fat 0 g Sodium 481 mg Potassium 129 mg Total carbohydrates 28 g Dietary fiber 0 g Sugars 24 g Protein 0 g

LEMON-LIME ELECTROLYTE DRINK

GOOD FOR: hydration • before, during, and after a workout

MAKES: 4¼ cups (1 liter) // **TIME:** 5 minutes to prep, plus resting overnight

You can use lemon juice, lime juice, or a combination of the two in this refreshing summer version of switchel. It tastes a lot like lemon-lime Gatorade.

Shake all the ingredients together, refrigerate overnight, strain, and drink.

4 cups (960 ml) water

2 tablespoons maple syrup

1 tablespoon apple cider vinegar

1 tablespoon fresh lime or lemon juice

¼ teaspoon sea salt, or to taste

3 SWITCHEL MOCKTAILS

Good for: hydration
Before and after a workout

These herbal-infused options are refreshing after a workout or even at a summer potluck! When you're forgoing alcohol to reach your fitness goals or support your health, these still feel festive.

Use the Lemon-Lime Electrolyte Drink recipe as the base for the following variations.

HERBED SWITCHEL

Add ¼ cup (5 g) basil or mint leaves, roughly torn, before refrigerating. Basil is naturally anti-inflammatory, while mint soothes an upset stomach—and it's refreshingly cool.

GROWN-UP KOOL-AID SWITCHEL

Add 2 tablespoons dried hibiscus flowers and ¼ cup (60 ml) orange juice before refrigerating. Hibiscus' sour, fruity flavor makes this taste like grown-up Kool-Aid! It's rich in vitamin C and is great for heart health.

THE GREYHOUND SWITCHEL

Add ¼ cup (60 ml) grapefruit juice and 1 tablespoon chopped fresh rosemary before refrigerating. Rosemary is invigorating and good for the memory, while grapefruit will help with dry mouth. If you're a fan of the taste of gin, add some crushed juniper berries for a drink reminiscent of a Greyhound. (You can also salt the rim of your glass.)

SWITCHEL SPORTS DRINKS WITH JUICE

GOOD FOR: hydration and carb replenishment • before, during, and after a workout

MAKES: about 5¼ cups (1.25 L) // **TIME:** 5 minutes to prep, plus resting overnight

These versions are sweeter for those who want to mask the taste of the vinegar. They're also higher in carbs, making them fuel as well as an electrolyte drink. We think these taste a lot like the ubiquitous sports drinks we all drank as kids!

4 cups (960 ml) water

1 cup (240 ml) juice (see suggestions below)

2 tablespoons apple cider vinegar

2 tablespoons maple syrup

¼ teaspoon sea salt, or to taste

Shake all the ingredients together, refrigerate overnight, and drink.

GRAPE: 1 cup (240 ml) grape juice (adds 140 calories, 38 g carbs)

FRUIT PUNCH: 1 cup (240 ml) fruit punch (adds 60 calories, 15 g carbs)

ORANGE: ½ cup (120 ml) fresh-squeezed orange juice and ½ cup (120 ml) white grape juice (fresh orange juice tastes less acidic than store-bought; adds 125 calories, 32 g carbs)

VERY BERRY: ½ cup (120 ml) white grape juice and ½ cup (120 ml) cranberry, blueberry, or raspberry juice blend (adds 130 calories, 34 g carbs)

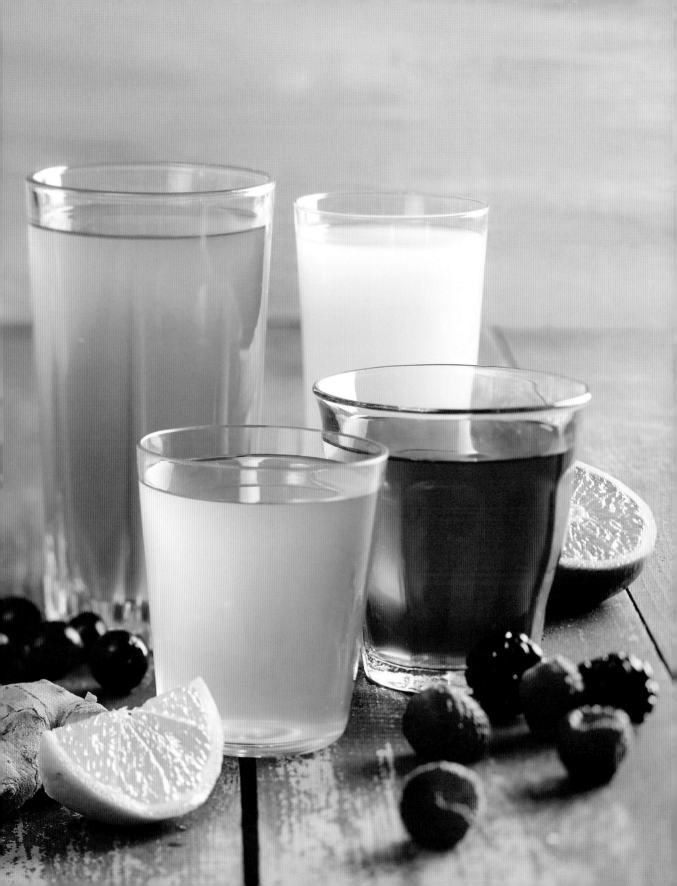

CUCUMBER-LIME ELECTROLYTE DRINK

GOOD FOR: hydration • before, during, and after a workout

MAKES: about 4¼ cups (1 L) // **TIME:** 5 minutes to prep, plus resting overnight

This refreshing, mildly sweet drink was inspired by the cult favorite flavor of Gatorade called Limon Pepino (Lime-Cucumber), part of a specialty Latino-focused line that's not distributed nationwide. We serendipitously discovered this drink at a bodega in downtown Cincinnati after a bike ride. It's cooling and sweet, and we're both thrilled and slightly disappointed that the hunt is over.

4 cups (960 ml) water

¼ cup (50 g) chopped cucumber

2 tablespoons maple syrup

1 tablespoon apple cider vinegar

1 tablespoon fresh lime juice

¼ teaspoon sea salt, or to taste

Shake all the ingredients together, refrigerate overnight, strain, and drink.

CRANBERRY-CITRUS ELECTROLYTE DRINK

GOOD FOR: hydration • before, during, and after a workout

MAKES: 5⅓ cups (1.3 L) // **TIME:** 5 minutes to prep, plus resting overnight

This version was inspired by a mention of *Sex and the City* while Stepf was listening to a podcast on a run. For those (like Matt) who haven't seen the show, the main character was fond of cosmopolitans, the cocktail made with cranberry juice, vodka, orange liqueur, and lime juice.

Shake all the ingredients together, refrigerate overnight, strain, and drink.

NOTE: *For this recipe, unsweetened cranberry juice is a bit too sour, so you want it to be blended with sweeter juices. If you only have 100 percent pure cranberry juice at home, mix it with apple or white grape juice to achieve desired sweetness.*

4 cups (960 ml) water

1 cup cranberry juice blend

2 tablespoons maple syrup

2 tablespoons orange juice

1 tablespoon apple cider vinegar

1 tablespoon fresh lime juice

1 teaspoon fresh lemon juice

¼ teaspoon sea salt, or to taste

MISO-MAPLE ELECTROLYTE "BROTH"

GOOD FOR: hydration, winter workouts • during and after a workout

MAKES: about 2¼ cups (540 ml) // **TIME:** 5 minutes

Sometimes what it takes to keep you going during a long workout or race isn't more calories, but more comfort. If you're an all-weather outdoor athlete, this substantial, drinkable broth is for you. Store in a thermos or insulated water bottle, and drink it to warm your belly midway through your workout.

1 tablespoon maple syrup

1 tablespoon white miso

1 to 2 tablespoons lime juice, to taste

½ teaspoon minced fresh ginger or garlic, optional

2 cups (480 ml) hot but not boiling water

Whisk together the maple syrup and miso. Add the lime juice and ginger, if using. Add the hot water. Pour immediately into your thermos or water bottle.

Nutrition info (for the entire recipe; without ginger or garlic): Calories 95 Total fat 1 g Sodium 636 mg Potassium 117 mg Total carbohydrates 21 g Dietary fiber 1 g Sugars 14 g Protein 2 g

UMEBOSHI ELECTROLYTE DRINK

GOOD FOR: hydration • before, during, and after a workout

MAKES: about 2 cups (480 ml) // **TIME:** 5 minutes

We've become quite creative in attempts to create sports drinks that someone with a sugar-averse palate can tolerate during exercise. This is a good one for anyone who deals with dry mouth. The salty-sour umeboshi paste, made from pickled, salted Japanese sour plums, stimulates the salivary glands. This version is mild for those new to the ingredient, but you can add more umeboshi paste if you'd like (in that case, keep an eye on the sodium content to make sure it meets your needs for your workout). We use sugar here to allow the flavor of the umeboshi to come through, but you can use another sweetener, such as agave nectar. (You can find umeboshi paste in the Asian aisle of most supermarkets.)

Combine all the ingredients in a water bottle or a jar with a lid. Shake well, then drink.

NOTE: *You can also suck on whole ume plums (mind the pit!) if you really like the flavor. Just be sure to drink plenty of water, because they're quite salty.*

2 cups (480 ml) water

1½ tablespoons sugar

1 teaspoon umeboshi paste

Nutrition info (for the entire recipe): Calories 73 Total fat 0 g Sodium 340 mg Potassium 10 mg Total carbohydrates 18 g Dietary fiber 0 g Sugars 18 g Protein 0 g

BLUEPRINT: 15 FLAVORED PROTEIN POWDERS

Neither of us uses protein powder regularly, but when we do, we want it to be free of any weird additives or artificial ingredients. After all, we're usually consuming it when plant-based meals or "real" food are hard to come by (when traveling, for example).

Having seen the many varieties of protein powder out there (usually with lengthy lists of hard-to-pronounce ingredients), we decided to make our own plant-based versions—all using real herbs, spices, and fruits! Once you know the blueprint these are based on, you customize your blends based on your palate and pantry.

For overnight hikes or long runs, you can add coconut or soy milk powder to your base formula, then shake with water when you're ready to drink.

1 Start with 4 servings store-bought plain protein powder. (With our variety, this was approximately 1 cup/85 g total protein powder.) Place your protein powder in a pint-size (500 ml) jar with a tight-fitting lid. Add the ingredients for one of the recipes listed below and shake well to combine. For items such as freeze-dried fruit, use the flat blade for dry ingredients on a mini blender.

2 Store your homemade protein powders in a cool, dark place (like your pantry) for up to 3 months.

NOTES:

These recipes are unsweetened. We prefer to sweeten smoothies naturally with bananas or dates. If you want to presweeten your protein powders, we recommend coconut sugar or a less-processed sugar. You'll want to grind it in the blender with the other ingredients.

To help prevent clumping, use a dry-blade grinder on a blender to combine with the protein powder.

VANILLA

1 tablespoon vanilla bean powder

CHOCOLATE

¼ cup (20 g) unsweetened cocoa
powder

CAPPUCCINO

1 tablespoon instant coffee

1 teaspoon vanilla bean powder

COFFEE

1 tablespoon instant coffee

GREEN TEA

1 tablespoon plus 1 teaspoon
matcha
(finely ground green tea)

STRAWBERRY

½ cup (15 g) freeze-dried
strawberries,
finely ground in a blender

TROPICAL

½ cup (30 g) freeze-dried
pineapple, finely ground in a
blender

¼ cup (20 g) unsweetened
shredded coconut, finely
ground in a blender

VANILLA CHAI

1 tablespoon unsweetened
shredded coconut, finely
ground in a blender

1 teaspoon vanilla bean powder

¼ teaspoon ground cardamom

¼ teaspoon ground cinnamon

⅛ teaspoon black pepper

SUPER FRUITS

¼ cup (25 g) "super fruit" powder
such as acai, pomegranate, and/
or goji

AMARETTO

1 tablespoon almond extract

PEANUT BUTTER CUP

¼ cup (25 g) powdered peanut
butter

2 tablespoons unsweetened cocoa
powder

MINT CHOCOLATE CHIP

¼ cup (20 g) unsweetened cocoa
powder

1 to 2 tablespoons dried mint,
finely ground in a blender

Note: This will be quite minty.
If you use mint you've dried
yourself, especially if it's
peppermint, it will be more
potent.

GERMAN CHOCOLATE

¼ cup (20 g) unsweetened
shredded coconut,
finely ground in a blender

2 tablespoons unsweetened cocoa
powder

¼ teaspoon almond extract

Note: Try adding cherries to your
smoothie when you make this
one!

MOCHA

2 tablespoons unsweetened cocoa
powder

1 tablespoon plus 1 teaspoon
instant coffee

PB&J

¼ cup (15 g) freeze-dried
strawberries,
finely ground in a blender

¼ cup (25 g) powdered peanut
butter

SOURCING INFO:

*Vanilla bean powder is simply dried, powdered vanilla bean seeds. You can find
it in the spice aisle.*

*Freeze-dried fruit is usually found in the bulk section next to the dried fruit.
You can use dried fruit instead, but it will not blend as well. For best results,
combine it with your protein powder before grinding.*

Tip: There's no reason
to suffer through gross-
tasting smoothies for
the sake of consuming
supplements or superfoods
like wheatgrass or spirulina.
Instead, pour your
smoothie into a glass, then
add about ¼ cup (60 ml)
water to the blender along
with your supplements.
Give it a whirl, then pour
into a small glass. Drink it
quickly, then wash it down
with your smoothie.

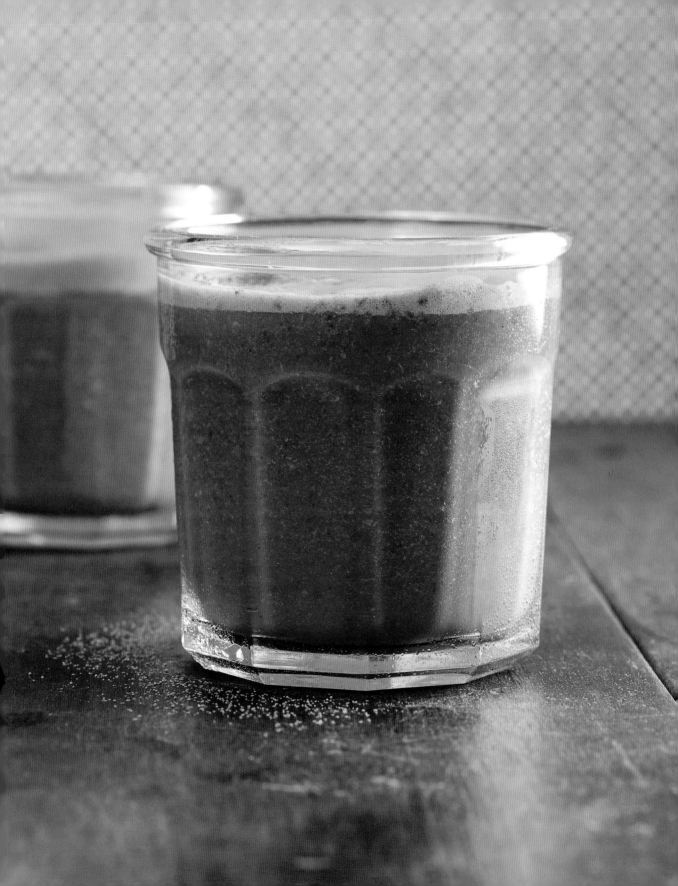

FROZEN MATCHA LATTE

GOOD FOR: recovery • after a workout

MAKES: 1 latte // **TIME:** 10 minutes

A Chinatown teahouse inspired this recipe, and once we tried using matcha in a smoothie, we were sold. Even with less sugar than a teahouse version, this drink still tastes like a frozen green tea latte. Want even more nutrition? Scoop ½ cup (115 g) Sweet Red Beans (page 253) into the bottom of the glass first. (That's how the original was served, and it was actually called a Shrek Shake.)

Combine all the ingredients in a high-speed blender until smooth and drink.

1 cup (240 ml) vanilla almond milk

1 cup (30 g) spinach or (15 g) kale, optional, for added color and nutrition

½ to 1 cup (70 to 140 g) ice

1 frozen ripe banana, in chunks for ease of blending

1 scoop vanilla protein powder, optional

2 teaspoons matcha powder

⅛ teaspoon vanilla bean powder

Nutrition info (with spinach and protein powder): Calories 320 Total fat 4 g Sodium 315 mg Potassium 798 mg Total carbohydrates 57 g Dietary fiber 7 g Sugars 31 g Protein 18 g

MARGARITA RECOVERY DRINK

GOOD FOR: recovery • after a workout

MAKES: 1 smoothie // **TIME:** 2 to 3 minutes

This smoothie is for those times you're out running in the heat, just dreaming of what cold, refreshing drink you'll have when you get home. Since a margarita will do nothing for your recovery (even if does sound pretty great when you're sweating buckets), we decided to capture the flavors of this cocktail favorite and turn them into a recovery smoothie. We recommend using citrus-, vanilla-, or berry-flavored protein powder, though it's just fine without. You can also substitute grapefruit juice for the orange. Try it with the salted or sugared rim on page 205.

1 cup (140 g) ice

1 cup (240 ml) water

¼ cup (60 ml) fresh lime juice (from 2 limes)

2 tablespoons orange juice

4 dates, pitted

1 scoop protein powder, optional

1 teaspoon coconut oil (OF: coconut milk)

Combine all the ingredients (except the ice if you want to serve this on the rocks) in a blender until smooth. Serve however you like your margaritas!

Tip: Ever get an upset stomach after chugging a smoothie? It might be your digestive system rebelling because you skipped that crucial first step: chewing! The three main sets of salivary glands each release an enzyme that breaks down fat, protein, or carbohydrates. By gulping down your smoothie, you're not giving those enzymes time to do their job. This smoothie is thick enough to eat with a spoon, which will slow you down a bit. But if your smoothie is sippable, swish it around your mouth a few times before swallowing. Your digestive system is already put through the wringer during a workout when much of your blood is needed elsewhere, so give it a break after your sweat session is over.

Nutrition info (with protein powder): Calories 251 Total fat 5 g Sodium 142 mg Potassium 322 mg Total carbohydrates 33 g Dietary fiber 5 g Sugars 24 g Protein 16 g

BULKED-UP SMOOTHIE

GOOD FOR: recovery • after a workout

MAKES: 1 smoothie // **TIME:** 2 to 3 minutes, not including time to cook beans

Want more protein in your smoothie without relying on powders or processed ingredients? Turn to our favorite plant-based food trio: a grain, a green, and a bean. Sound weird in a smoothie? Not to worry—it tastes great (like a chocolate–peanut butter smoothie), thanks to all the other ingredients involved. The trick here is to use plain cooked beans, preferably salt-free. (Leftover cumin-flavored beans might not blend in so well!) Omit the berries and this shake will taste like the old "weight-gainer" shakes you may remember fondly from your younger days.

Combine all the ingredients in a high-speed blender and drink.

3 cups (85 g) mixed baby greens

1 cup (240 ml) almond milk

1 cup (140 g) ice, optional

½ cup (100 g) cooked cannellini, adzuki, or black beans

½ cup (75 g) berries, optional

¼ cup (24 g) GF old-fashioned rolled oats

1 banana

2 tablespoons almond butter

1 tablespoon unsweetened cocoa powder

Nutrition info (with berries): Calories 712 Total fat 26 g Sodium 463 mg Potassium 1,957 mg Total carbohydrates 105 g Dietary fiber 24 g Sugars 37 g Protein 29 g

LEAN GREEN SMOOTHIE

GOOD FOR: recovery • after a workout

MAKES: 1 smoothie // **TIME:** 2 to 3 minutes

Do you find most smoothies to be too sweet for your taste? If so, then you'll love this one. It's as slimmed-down as can be, in both calories and sweetness. The banana binds the almond milk and greens; without something creamy they would separate and create an unappealing texture. This is a great smoothie to highlight a particular herb or spice. Try cinnamon, which can help stabilize your blood sugar, or turmeric and ginger to fight inflammation.

3 cups (85 g) mixed baby greens

1 cup (240 ml) almond milk

1 small ripe banana

Protein powder, optional

Assorted herbs and spices:
1 tablespoon minced fresh ginger, 1 teaspoon minced fresh turmeric, 1 teaspoon ground cinnamon, ¼ teaspoon vanilla bean powder, 1 tablespoon unsweetened cocoa powder, 1 tablespoon maca powder, etc.

Combine all the ingredients in a blender and drink.

Nutrition info (with protein powder, without herbs or spices): Calories 302 Total fat 5 g Sodium 570 mg Potassium 1,281 mg Total carbohydrates 40 g Dietary fiber 9 g Sugars 16 g Protein 22 g

MATT'S KID-FRIENDLY EVERYDAY DOUBLE BERRY BANANA SMOOTHIE

GOOD FOR: fuel • before a workout

MAKES: 2 smoothies // **TIME:** 2 to 3 minutes

As athletic goals have gradually given way to the priorities and time constraints that come along with having children, Matt's go-to smoothie has transformed into one that can be made quickly. And, it's a smoothie that the kids enjoy day in and day out, despite taste buds that seem to change with the day of the week. Make it more superfood-y as desired; we often include a tablespoon or so of wheatgrass powder and goji berries to get more nutrition in the glass without sacrificing taste.

Combine all the ingredients in a blender and serve.

3 cups (720 ml) water

3 ripe (spotted!) bananas

1 cup (140 g) frozen raspberries

1 cup (150 g) frozen strawberries

A big handful or two of baby spinach or other mild-tasting greens, optional

2 tablespoons ground flaxseeds or chia seeds

2 tablespoons raw walnuts

Nutrition info (for the entire recipe; without greens): Calories 619 Total fat 18 g Sodium 13 mg Potassium 1,977 mg Total carbohydrates 118 g Dietary fiber 26 g Sugars 59 g Protein 13 g

FUN WAYS
to Garnish Your Smoothies

Smoothies are a way of life for a No Meat Athlete, but they can lose their appeal rather quickly during training season. We know that you may not need a "recipe" for a smoothie at this stage in your training, but you *do* need some fun toppings and add-ons to help liven up your daily habit!

Our chocolate "magic shell" is similar to the coating on dipped ice cream cones, without all the weird ingredients. Thanks to the unique characteristics of coconut oil, the shell will harden when it hits the ice-cold smoothie but melt as soon as it touches your tongue. If your smoothie is thick enough to eat with a spoon, go for it—you'll feel like you're eating dessert!

The salted or sugared hempseed rim was inspired by the Buchi-rita at the Buchi Bar in Asheville. They mix spicy kombucha with tequila and serve it with the same salty, crunchy rim. It added such a unique touch that we started adding it to juices at home, along with sugar and citrus zest. These little touches can make a big difference, especially when you're skipping alcohol and treats during training.

Chocolate Magic Shell

1 tablespoon coconut oil
(OF: swap coconut butter, but it will not set as solidly or melt quite as much)

2 teaspoons chocolate chips

1 Microwave the coconut oil and chocolate chips in a small ramekin until the chocolate chips begin to melt, 15 to 30 seconds. (You can also use a small saucepan on the stove over medium-low heat.) Stir to combine and allow residual heat to finish melting the chocolate. Set aside.

2 Scoop one quarter of the smoothie into a large glass or canning jar, then drizzle with about 1 teaspoon of the coconut-chocolate mixture. Repeat with the remaining smoothie and coconut-chocolate mixture. The cold smoothie will instantly freeze the chocolaty coconut oil into a crispy "shell" that will make your shake seem like dessert. Eat with a spoon immediately.

Salted or Sugared Hempseed Rim

SALTED

1 tablespoon hemp seeds

1 tablespoon lime, lemon, or orange zest

1 teaspoon coarse salt

1 teaspoon raw sugar

SUGARED

1 tablespoon hemp seeds

1 tablespoon lime, lemon, or orange zest

1 teaspoon maple syrup

1 teaspoon raw sugar

Pinch of coarse salt

Mix all the ingredients on a small saucer. Moisten the top of your glass and dip into the hemp mixture. Pour in your beverage and enjoy.

Building a Smoothie Bowl

Smoothie bowls are all the rage these days. If you really want to savor every ounce of a smoothie, scale back on the liquid or use mostly frozen fruit, then pour it into a bowl. (This can also help ward off the bellyache that can happen when you chug your smoothie!) Top as desired, with these suggestions or your own ideas:

Granola, buckwheat groats, or whole-grain cereal

Fresh berries, sliced banana or peaches, or diced mango

Shredded coconut, dried or freeze-dried fruit, or cacao nibs

Nut butter or chopped nuts and seeds such as ground flaxseed or hemp seeds (We don't recommend chia here, since it should be soaked in water to avoid abdominal discomfort.)

TROPICAL VACATION RECOVERY SMOOTHIE

GOOD FOR: recovery • after a workout

MAKES: 1 smoothie // **TIME:** 5 minutes

Some training days are harder than others, and we've all had those workouts where you wish you could throw in the towel and relax on the beach instead of sweating it out. This smoothie is the perfect antidote to a lackluster performance. Every sip tastes like a day at the beach, but it's working behind the scenes to fight inflammation, thanks to the inclusion of pineapple.

1 cup (165 g) frozen pineapple

1 cup (240 ml) light coconut milk

½ cup (120 ml) orange juice

½ cup (120 ml) pineapple juice

Protein powder, optional

Toasted coconut

Combine the pineapple, coconut milk, orange juice, pineapple juice, and protein powder, if using, in a blender. Garnish with the toasted coconut and serve.

Nutrition info (with protein powder): Calories 457 Total fat 15 g Sodium 76 mg Potassium 1,077 mg Total carbohydrates 69 g Dietary fiber 13 g Sugars 51 g Protein 18 g

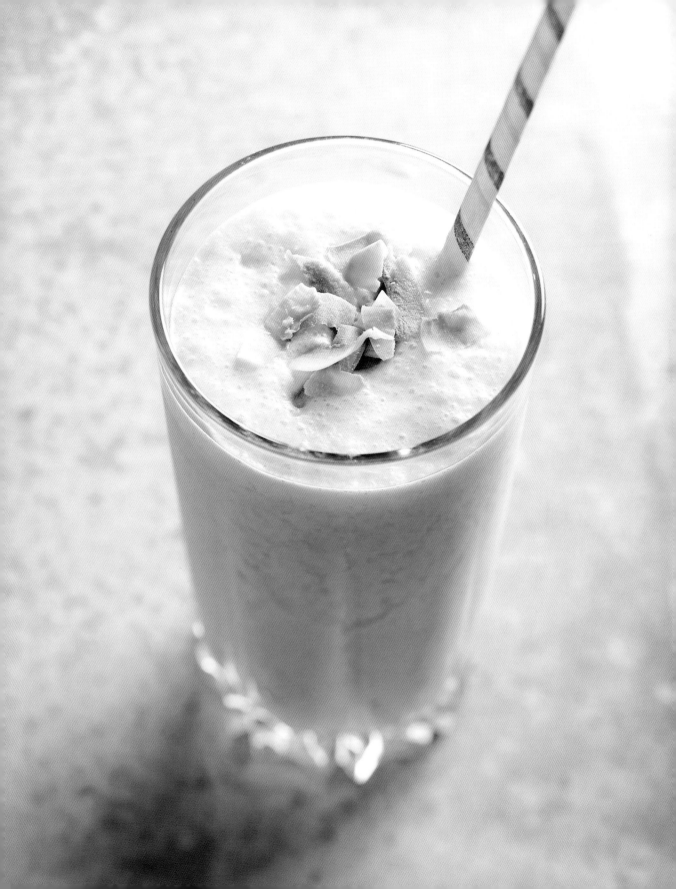

BAN THE BLOAT DANDELION-PINEAPPLE SMOOTHIE

GOOD FOR: recovery • after a workout

MAKES: 1 smoothie // **TIME:** 2 to 3 minutes

Ever feel bloated and sluggish the day (or days) after an extra-long run or race? That swelling is inflammation, and while it's there to help protect your body as part of your natural defense system, it certainly doesn't feel good. Enter this smoothie, packed full of nutritious, unusual-but-delicious ingredients designed to help fight inflammation and banish the bloat. (It's also really good after air travel or an indulgent vacation.)

Dandelions are a natural diuretic, which means they help expel excess water from the body. Combined with water to help flush out your system, this drink is more like a thick, whole food juice than a smoothie. Without a creamy component to bind the ingredients together it can start to separate, so drink it quickly or serve in a blender bottle to easily remix it.

2 cups (110 g) dandelion greens (about 4 to 6 stems)

1 orange, peeled, separated into segments, and seeds removed

1 to 2 cups (240 to 480 ml) water

1 cup (165 g) fresh or frozen pineapple chunks

1-inch (2.5 cm) piece ginger (no need to peel)

2 tablespoons fresh lime juice

½ to 1 teaspoon ground turmeric (see Note)

Combine all the ingredients in a blender, adding water as needed to reach desired consistency. Drink immediately.

NOTE: *Start with the smaller amount of turmeric, then add more to taste.*

Nutrition info: Calories 270 Total fat 2 g Sodium 89 mg Potassium 1,044 mg Total carbohydrates 67 g Dietary fiber 10 g Sugars 45 g Protein 6 g

V9

GOOD FOR: carb replenishment • after a workout

MAKES: 2 smoothies // **TIME:** 10 minutes

Take your veggies and go! This smoothie is for those who prefer savory to sweet. It's, of course, a play on the popular vegetable juice. Serve chilled in a glass with a salted celery–hemp seed rim and all the trimmings you'd use in a Bloody Mary. If there's a veggie you don't like, leave it out or add more of another.

1 Combine the spinach, tomatoes, carrots, celery, bell pepper, beet, parsley, scallion, basil, cayenne, and celery seed in a high-speed blender. Process, adding enough water and ice to achieve desired texture. Strain if desired.

2 Pour into glasses and serve, garnishing with additional parsley or basil.

Variation: Turn this into a light meal by pouring into a bowl and garnishing with sunflower seeds, a drizzle of olive oil (or tahini), and a smattering of chopped lettuce.

2 cups (60 g) spinach or (30 g) kale

2 tomatoes, cored

2 large carrots, roughly chopped

1 celery rib, roughly chopped (keep the leaves if there are any)

1 red or yellow bell pepper, cored and roughly chopped

1 small beet, peeled and cubed

Handful flat-leaf parsley leaves, plus more for garnish

1 scallion (white and light green parts), sliced

3 large basil leaves, plus more for garnish

Pinch cayenne pepper

Pinch celery seed

1 to 2 cups (240 to 480 ml) water

½ to 1 cup (70 to 140 g) ice

Nutrition info (for the entire recipe): Calories 171 Total fat 1 g Sodium 214 mg Potassium 1265 mg Total carbohydrates 36 g Dietary fiber 12 g Sugars 22 g Protein 7 g

OFO XS GF FF

BETTER THAN BONE BROTH

GOOD FOR: recovery, hydration, winter workouts • after a workout

MAKES: 2 quarts (2 L) broth // **TIME:** At least 8 hours or overnight

Bone broth is all the rage, so we thought we'd create a plant-based version that trumps it. No bones about it—or *in* it—this broth is packed with nutrients. Instead of focusing on the "bone-building benefits" of bone broth, we turned our attention to the benefits of a mushroom-based broth. The immune-boosting properties of mushrooms are well documented, and we wanted to create a broth that could stand on its own or be used as the base for another recipe. Maitake (hen of the woods) mushrooms support normal cell growth and have been studied for their immunostimulating properties. They are available dried and fresh in most large supermarkets. (But if you can't find them, feel free to swap in your favorite "wild" mushroom blend.)

Reishi is an optional ingredient here, but if you can find it, it's well worth including. This medicinal mushroom has been used in China and Japan for centuries. It has been studied for its antioxidant, immunosupportive, and anticancer properties. You only need a bit, and you can reuse your dried reishi a few times—that's how potent it is! Head to your local co-op or health food store for this one.

The medicinal 'shrooms called for here are good for the immune system, and they also get attention for being adaptogens, meaning they help our bodies respond to stress.

1 tablespoon olive oil (OF: ¼ cup/60 ml water)

1 onion, roughly chopped

2 celery ribs, chopped

1 carrot, chopped

3 garlic cloves, chopped

One 10-ounce (283 g) package cremini mushrooms, trimmed and sliced

1 ounce (25 g) dried shiitake mushrooms, broken into pieces, or 1 pint fresh shiitakes, sliced

1 ounce (25 g) dried maitake mushrooms, or 1 bunch fresh, roughly chopped

1-inch (2.5 cm) piece dried reishi mushroom, optional

1 Heat the oil in a slow cooker set to high or a pressure cooker. (You can also use the sauté setting on an Instant Pot/pressure cooker.)

2 Add the onion, celery, carrot, garlic, and cremini. Cook, stirring occasionally, until fragrant and the vegetables start to get some color, about 10 minutes.

3 Add the shiitakes and maitakes to the slow cooker. (If using fresh shiitake or maitake mushrooms, allow them to cook until starting soften and release juices, about 2 minutes, before continuing with the recipe. If using dried, simply add them to the slow cooker and proceed with the next step.)

4 Add the reishi, if using. Add the water, place the lid on the slow cooker, and cook on low for 1 day, checking the water level every few hours.

5 Remove the reishi and reserve for additional use(s). Strain the broth and, if desired, reserve the vegetables (see Tip). Season with salt and pepper to taste.

6 Pour into quart-size (1 L) jars. Let cool slightly, and refrigerate for up to 4 days or freeze (leaving ½-inch/1.25 cm head space in jars) for up to 3 months.

> **Tip:** Don't throw away those leftover veggies; instead, turn them into a quick mushroom "pâté." Puree them in a food processor along with a bit of Cashew Cream (page 236), plenty of fresh parsley, and salt and pepper to taste. Spread on toast or use as a veggie dip.

8 cups (2 L) water

Salt and black pepper

Nutrition info (for the entire recipe): Calories 375 Total fat 15 g Sodium 77 mg Potassium 1,870 mg Total carbohydrates 56 g Dietary fiber 11 g Sugars 16 g Protein 15 g

OF: 255 calories, 1 g fat

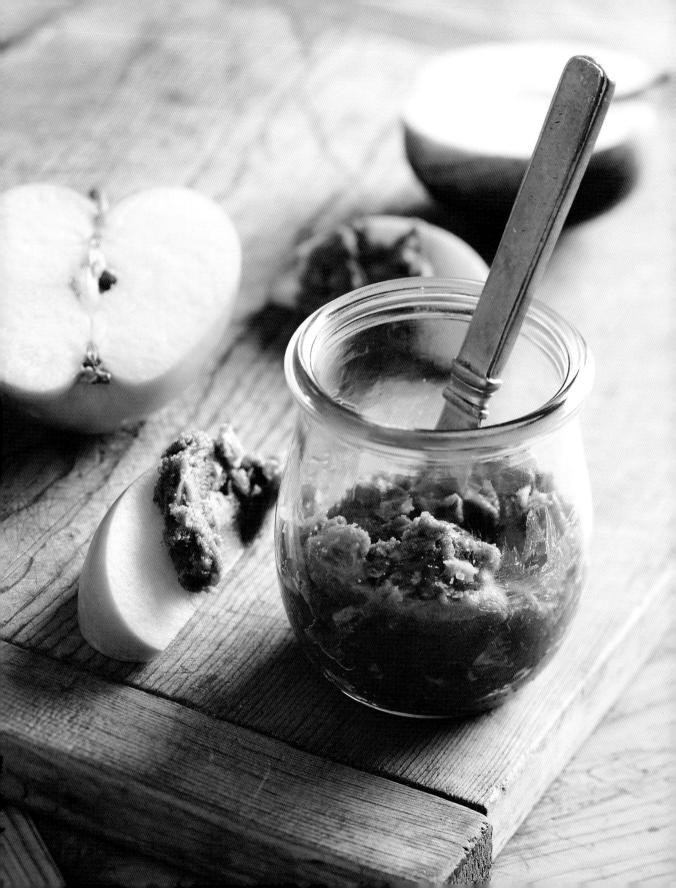

PIÑA COLADA ALMOND BUTTER

GOOD FOR: fuel • during and after a workout

SERVES: 6 to 8 // **TIME:** 5 minutes

Packets of flavored nut butters are quick, easy fuel, so we created a tropical version that'll give you something to look forward to on those extra long days when you need more than just carbohydrates to get you through the workout or race. (There's about 6 grams of protein, 8 grams of carbs, and 18 grams of fat per 2 tablespoons.) This almond butter is a beach vacation in the middle of a suffer fest. While it's perfect fuel for when you're on the go, it's also great spread on apple slices or toast.

Thoroughly combine all the ingredients in a small bowl. To take it on the go, put each serving in parchment paper, then inside a ziplock bag. Tear a small hole in the parchment, then suck out the almond butter as desired (it's thick enough that it won't leak). The nut butter can be stored in a jar and refrigerated for up to 1 week. (Omit the coconut milk if you want to store it longer.)

½ cup (125 g) creamy almond (or cashew) butter

¼ cup (50 g) dried pineapple, minced

2 tablespoons unsweetened coconut flakes

1 to 2 tablespoons full-fat coconut milk

1 teaspoon sugar

Salt to taste (use more if your nut butter is unsalted; we used about ¼ teaspoon)

Nutrition info (for the entire recipe): Calories 954 Total fat 71 g Sodium 769 mg Potassium 26 mg Total carbohydrates 61 g Dietary fiber 14 g Sugars 40 g Protein 25 g

SESAME-TAMARI PORTABLE RICE BALLS

GOOD FOR: fuel • during a workout

MAKES: 18 rice balls // **TIME:** 20 minutes to prep, 25 minutes to cook

A while back, the concept of "portables"—aka on-the-bike fuel made in your own kitchen with quick-burning carbs like white rice—began floating around cycling and triathlon blogs. However, most of them contained meat, cheese, or eggs, so those wouldn't work for us. Inspired by those recipes, as well as traditional Japanese rice balls (similar to what vegan ultramarathon legend Scott Jurek has in his book) and Korean "triangle sushi," we created several plant-based varieties. This is our favorite savory version.

Why white rice? You've likely noticed that we use whole grains almost exclusively throughout the book, yet here we opt for white rice. Typically, the fiber and other nutrients found in the bran of brown rice are desirable, but during a workout they just slow down the amount of time it takes for your body to make use of the carbohydrates. White rice is better immediate fuel for your fire.

3 cups (720 ml) water

3 cups (540 g) white sushi rice, rinsed

½ cup (70 g) toasted white or black sesame seeds

2 tablespoons raw sugar

2 tablespoons reduced-sodium GF tamari, or to taste

1 teaspoon ume plum or rice vinegar

1 tablespoon toasted sesame oil (OF: omit)

1 Bring the water to a boil in a large saucepan, then lower the heat to medium-low and stir in the rice. Cook, stirring often, until soft, about 15 to 20 minutes. You want it to be moist (but not soggy) and very sticky and tender.

2 Transfer the cooked rice to a large bowl. Working quickly, add all but 2 tablespoons of the sesame seeds, the sugar, tamari, and vinegar. Stir thoroughly to combine and allow to cool slightly.

3 Wet your hands to prevent the rice from sticking. Scoop about ½ cup (100 g) of the rice mixture into your hands. Form a ball, applying gentle but firm pressure. Repeat with the remaining rice; let sit for 5 minutes.

4 Brush the rice balls with the sesame oil, sprinkle with the remaining 2 tablespoons sesame seeds, and wrap in plastic wrap or parchment paper. Refrigerate for up to 1 week or freeze individual rice balls for up to 3 months. (If frozen, allow to thaw overnight before eating.)

Nutrition info (for the entire recipe): Calories 3,066 Total fat 50 g Sodium 1,588 mg Potassium 337 mg Total carbohydrates 606 g Dietary fiber 24 g Sugars 27 g Protein 81 g

GREEN ENERGY BITES

GOOD FOR: fuel • before, during, and after a workout

MAKES: 36 energy bites // **TIME:** 15 minutes to prep

The distinct flavor of spirulina is somehow masked in this simple energy bite—and that's no easy feat! Inspired by the green bites sold in bulk at health-food stores, these chunks are intended for on-the-go snacking and mid-race fueling.

Spirulina is blue-green algae that's incredibly high in protein (by weight). More than 60 percent of it is protein! In lab studies, it has been shown to boost probiotic growth. It can absorb undesirable heavy metals from the water where it grows, so choose a reliable source that tests for such things.

1 Pulse the dates in a food processor until they form a paste. Add the sunflower seeds and cashews. Pulse until roughly chopped, then add the carob and spirulina. Pulse a couple of times, then process until thoroughly combined.

2 Transfer to a rectangular glass dish (we used a 6-cup/1.4 L glass storage container) lined with parchment paper. Press down, using a small piece of parchment to keep your fingers from sticking to the bars. Sprinkle with the coconut and salt.

3 Pull the parchment out of the container and slice into 36 pieces. Store in an airtight container for up to 1 week or freeze for up to 3 months.

1½ cups (220 g) pitted dates, soaked in hot water for 5 minutes and drained

½ cup (75 g) raw sunflower seeds

½ cup (60 g) roasted, unsalted cashews

¼ cup (40 g) carob or chocolate chips

2 tablespoons spirulina powder or another greens powder

2 tablespoons unsweetened shredded coconut

Pinch of salt

Nutrition info (for the entire recipe): Calories 1,729 Total fat 79 g Sodium 6 mg Potassium 1,951 mg Total carbohydrates 231 g Dietary fiber 18 g Sugars 160 g Protein 33 g

STRAWBERRY SHORTCAKE RICE BITES

GOOD FOR: fuel • before, during, and after a workout

MAKES: 6 to 8 rolls // **TIME:** 20 minutes to prep, 25 minutes to cook

As we created more varieties of portable fuel, we discovered that certain ingredients didn't lend themselves well to the "rice ball" shape. We wanted to integrate fruit, but it was messy, so we decided to create some sushi-style rolls, sliced for easy eating on the go. These Strawberry Shortcake bites are sweet and slightly tangy. The "shortcake" flavor comes from the vanilla; the vanilla also gives the sushi rice a flavor similar to rice pudding. Feel free to swap in another berry or soft fruit, if desired.

3 cups (720 ml) water

3 cups (540 g) white sushi rice

½ cup (100 g) raw sugar, or to taste

3 tablespoons fresh lemon juice

½ teaspoon vanilla extract

2 cups (1 pint/290 g) strawberries, hulled and quartered

3 tablespoons chia seeds

Salt, optional

1 Bring the water to a boil in a large saucepan, then lower the heat to medium-low and stir in the rice. Cook, stirring often, until soft, about 15 to 20 minutes. You want it to be moist (but not soggy) and very sticky and tender.

2 Transfer the cooked rice to a large bowl. Working quickly, add the sugar, lemon juice, and vanilla. Stir thoroughly to combine and allow to cool slightly.

3 Spread out a sushi mat or silicone liner. Cover with plastic wrap and spread 1 cup (195 g) rice on top of the plastic. With wet hands, press the rice into a uniform ½-inch (13 mm) thick layer.

4 Place a row of strawberries, end to end, about 1 inch (2.5 cm) from the bottom edge. Sprinkle with 1 teaspoon chia seeds. Starting with the edge closest to you, roll the rice tightly into a cylinder, using the plastic wrap and mat to assist. Be sure to pull the plastic and mat away from the rice as you roll. Repeat with the remaining ingredients.

5 Sprinkle the outside of the rolls with salt to taste, if desired. Let sit for 5 minutes, then slice each roll into 8 to 10 pieces using a very sharp knife. Wrap tightly in parchment paper and plastic wrap if eating on the go. Refrigerate for up to 2 days or freeze individual pieces for up to 3 months. (If frozen, allow to thaw overnight before eating.)

NOTE: *We generally dislike using plastic, but it does help these rice bites hold together better than parchment alone.*

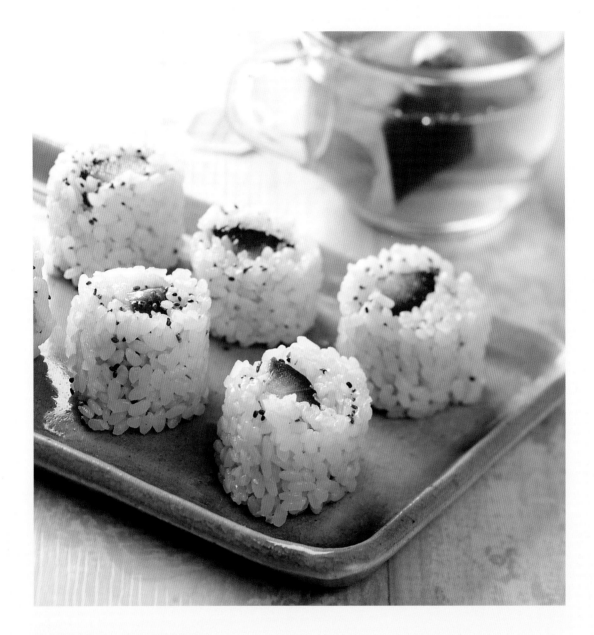

Variation: For Key Lime Pie Rice Bites, swap in lime juice for the lemon, omit the strawberries, and stir in 2 tablespoons full-fat coconut milk as well as an additional tablespoon of chia. Refrigerate for up to 1 week, or freeze individual pieces for up to 3 months. Thaw overnight, then take on your workout.

Nutrition info (for the entire Strawberry Shortcake recipe; without salt): Calories 3,081 Total fat 13 g Sodium 199 mg Potassium 517 mg Total carbohydrates 699 g Dietary fiber 34 g Sugars 116 g Protein 72 g

Nutrition info (for the entire Key Lime Pie recipe): Calories 2,983 Total fat 12 g Sodium 196 mg Potassium 52 mg Total carbohydrates 675 g Dietary fiber 28 g Sugars 101 g Protein 70 g

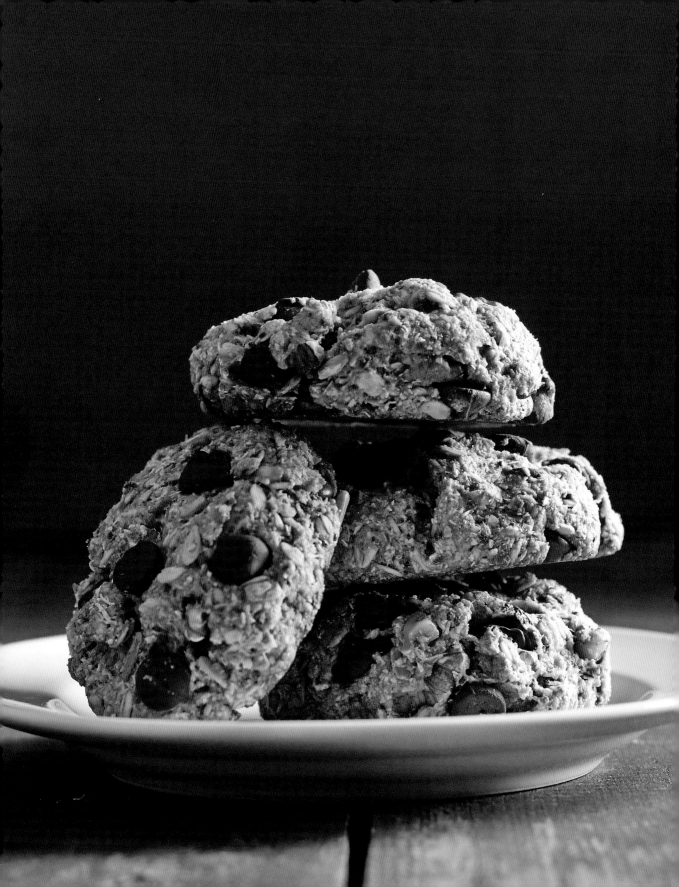

CALORIE BOMB COOKIES

GOOD FOR: fuel • before (as treat), during, and after (as treat) a workout

MAKES: 12 giant cookies (or 24 regular cookies) // **TIME:** 15 minutes to prep, 30 minutes to bake

These cookies fueled the BSM cycling team (cofounded by Stepf's husband, Sam) through a ten-hour road trip and epic adventure ride a few summers back. They're hefty yet easy to eat and digest in the saddle or driver's seat; they're also packed with as much real food and as many calories as possible, hence the name.

1 Preheat the oven to 350°F (180°C). Line two baking sheets with parchment paper.

2 Place 2 cups (195 g) of the oats in a food processor or blender and pulse until they are finely ground. Transfer to a large bowl and add the flour, baking powder, salt, and remaining oats.

3 Combine the bananas, sugar, oil, water, chia seeds, and vanilla in the blender or food processor. Add to the oat mixture and stir with a sturdy wooden spoon until combined. Add the chocolate chips, walnuts, sunflower seeds, and coconut.

4 With wet hands, form about ½ cup (60 g) dough into balls for giant cookies, about ¼ cup (30 g) dough for regular cookies. (There should be 6 balls on each baking sheet if making giant cookies.) Flatten them to ¾ to 1 inch (2 to 2.5 cm) thick.

5 Bake for 30 minutes, or until golden brown. Allow to cool completely before removing from the baking sheets. Store in an airtight container for up to 1 week or freeze for up to 3 months. Wrap in parchment paper for on-the-go eating.

Variations: Use coconut extract in place of the vanilla. Swap carob for the chocolate. Dice mini peanut butter cups and add to the mix.

4 cups (385 g) old-fashioned rolled oats

1½ cups (225 g) whole wheat flour

1 teaspoon baking powder

½ teaspoon salt

3 ripe bananas

1 cup (200 g) raw sugar or coconut sugar

⅓ cup (80 ml) coconut oil (OF: coconut butter)

¼ cup plus 2 tablespoons (90 ml) water

2 tablespoons chia seeds or ground flaxseeds

2 teaspoons vanilla extract

1 cup (225 g) dark chocolate chips

1 cup (120 g) raw walnut pieces

½ cup (75 g) raw sunflower seeds

½ cup (40 g) unsweetened shredded coconut, optional

Nutrition info (for the entire recipe; with shredded coconut): Calories 5,893 Total fat 291 g Sodium 1,371 mg Potassium 2,471 mg Total carbohydrates 819 g Dietary fiber 97 g Sugars 359 g Protein 97 g

CHOCOLATE-COCONUT-PECAN CHEWY BARS

GOOD FOR: fuel • before, during, and after a workout

MAKES: 8 bars // **TIME:** 15 minutes to prep, 10 minutes to bake

These will remind you of seven-layer bars, but they're much faster to make, not to mention healthier (we hold the sweetened condensed milk, butter, and butterscotch). If your bars tend to melt in your jersey pocket in summer, leave these at home and reward yourself after the workout. In most locales, they can be mid-workout fuel the other three seasons of the year.

1 cup (150 g) pitted dates, soaked in hot water for 10 minutes and drained

¼ cup (60 ml) brown rice syrup

⅓ cup (40 g) plus ¼ cup (30 g) chopped pecans

1½ cups (145 g) old-fashioned rolled oats

⅓ cup (55 g) mini chocolate chips

⅓ cup (30 g) unsweetened shredded coconut

1. Preheat the oven to 300°F (150°C). Line a 9-inch (23 cm) square baking dish with parchment paper.

2. Pulse, then process the dates in a food processor until smooth. Transfer to a large bowl, then stir in the brown rice syrup.

3. Process ¼ cup (30 g) of the pecans and ½ cup (50 g) of the oats in the now-empty food processor until finely ground. Add to the bowl with the dates, then fold in the remaining pecans, remaining oats, the chocolate chips, and coconut. (The dates and syrup make this thick so you'll need to use some muscle to fold the ingredients.)

4. Transfer to the dish. Bake for 10 minutes, or until fragrant and golden brown. Allow to cool completely, then slice into 8 bars using a sharp knife and serve.

5. Store in an airtight container for up to 1 week. Individual bars can be wrapped in parchment and taken on the go.

Nutrition info (for the entire recipe): Calories 2,347 Total fat 81 g Sodium 295 mg Potassium 1,438 mg Total carbohydrates 407 g Dietary fiber 31 g Sugars 144 g Protein 26 g

Chapter 8

FLAVOR BOOSTS (SPICE BLENDS, SAUCES & OTHER TASTY ADD-ONS)

J ust as there's a tendency to move toward one-dish meals once you begin a plant-based diet, we've noticed it's also quite easy to fall into the trap of eating food that's nutritionally stellar but somewhat lackluster in the flavor department. (A certain unnamed spouse calls such meals "gruel.") However, there's no need to suffer through bland food while you're training or when you're short on time. Our simple sauces, spice blends, and tasty toppings can turn even the most mundane meal into something special.

Building in flavor is especially important if you're just starting out on this journey of adopting a plant-based diet and you're trying to develop new habits; you don't want to just "survive" your meals, the way too many people do on crash diets. As has been said many times: If it doesn't become a lifestyle, it's not going to last. And guess what? The only chance any diet has of becoming a lifestyle is if you genuinely enjoy the food you eat. Otherwise, every meal you eat represents a tiny drain on your willpower—and because habit change is a race to see if you can make something your new normal before your willpower runs out, you want to preserve every bit of it you can.

So don't take the lazy way out and force yourself to get through another meal just because it's healthy; you might hurt your chances of eating healthy for the long haul! With only a tiny bit of advance planning and time, you can throw together a few bold spice blends that will last you for months. Then whenever you want to dress up simple beans and rice or a basic stir-fry, all you've got to do is reach for a single jar in your spice cabinet. Or, you can whip up a sauce, dip, or topping that will turn your ho-hum dinner into a memorable meal. If you're the kind of person who cooks giant batches once a week, turn to this chapter as a way to avoid burnout when you're eating your sixth-consecutive serving of quinoa and roasted broccoli.

SPICE BLENDS

There are two reasons why restaurant meals frequently taste so much better than our home-cooked versions. First, chefs are often heavy-handed with the sugar, salt, and fat. But that trick is not going to help you meet your fitness goals! The second reason, however, can help you: Chefs also use liberal doses of herbs and spices. These are packed with phytochemicals that can support your well-being—and even speed up your recovery and combat inflammation in some cases.

You can buy jarred spice blends, but they often contain unnecessary sugar or salt, flow agents to prevent caking, and flavor enhancers (such as MSG and maltodextrin). We suggest making them yourself with the recipes in this section—these blends keep for a few months in your pantry and take only a few minutes to prepare. Keep costs down and spices fresh by buying the exact amounts you need from the bulk bins.

Just as whole foods are fresher and more flavorful than processed ones, the same is true of whole spices. When possible, choose whole over ground and grind them yourself. If you're substituting ground spices for whole, add an additional ¼ teaspoon or so for extra flavor.

GARAM MASALA

MAKES: about ½ cup (50 g) // **TIME:** 5 minutes

This blend of Indian spices translates to "hot mixture." While it's not spicy per se, it is warming for the body. Cardamom is sold both as seeds, which are black and what you want to use to cook, and pods, which are green and must be opened to get to the seeds. Buy either one, but be sure to discard the pods before grinding! You can use a mini blender with a flat blade instead of a coffee grinder. Use this potent blend in Indian recipes to add depth or on roasted vegetables. It can also be stirred into coconut yogurt with salt and lemon juice as a quick dip for Pakoras (page 165).

Pulse all the ingredients in a clean coffee grinder until thoroughly combined. Store in an airtight container for up to 6 months.

2 tablespoons black peppercorns

2 tablespoons coriander seeds

2 tablespoons cumin seeds

1 teaspoon freshly grated nutmeg or 1¼ teaspoons ground nutmeg

1 teaspoon ground cinnamon

1 teaspoon whole cloves

¼ teaspoon cardamom seeds

> **Tip:** Clean your coffee grinder by pulsing rice or coarse salt in it. Do not use water, as this will pick up all the oils left over from coffee or spices. Wipe clean with a lint-free towel or a dry brush.

ITALIAN SPICES

MAKES: about ½ cup (50 g) **//** **TIME:** 5 minutes

This simple, versatile blend pairs well with tomato sauce, seasons beans like a dream, and can be added to a vinaigrette, with or without oil.

¼ cup (15 g) dried oregano

3 tablespoons fennel seeds

1 tablespoon garlic powder

Shake all the ingredients together in a jar with a tight-fitting lid. Store for up to 6 months.

Variation: For spicy Italian seasoning, add 1 teaspoon crushed red pepper.

JERK SPICES

MAKES: about ⅓ cup (30 g) // **TIME:** 5 minutes

While the ingredient list for jerk seasoning is lengthy, the components are fairly common and the result is well worth the effort. A batch will keep for months, and this seasoning blend is versatile: Try it on roasted veggies, rub it onto tofu or tempeh, or stir it into jarred tomato sauce with a bit of coconut milk to serve on pasta or rice for a quick dinner.

Pulse all the ingredients in a clean coffee grinder until thoroughly combined. Store in an airtight container for up to 6 months.

1 tablespoon garlic powder

2 teaspoons dark brown sugar

2 teaspoons dried thyme

2 teaspoons onion powder

2 teaspoons salt, optional

1 teaspoon black pepper

1 teaspoon dried parsley

1 teaspoon sweet paprika

1 teaspoon whole allspice

½ teaspoon cayenne pepper

½ teaspoon crushed red pepper

¼ teaspoon cumin seeds

¼ teaspoon freshly grated nutmeg

¼ teaspoon ground cinnamon

> **Tip:** Turn this into a wet rub for tofu or tempeh by combining 2 tablespoons of the spice blend with 2 tablespoons grape jam or apple butter.

TACO SEASONING

MAKES: ½ cup (50 g) // **TIME:** 5 minutes

Skip those packets of taco seasoning: You're mostly paying for MSG and salt. Here, cumin, paprika, and chili powder are the main ingredients, and we omit the salt so you get to control the sodium level of your final dish.

3 tablespoons ground cumin

2 tablespoons chili powder

2 tablespoons sweet or smoked paprika

2 teaspoons dried oregano

1 teaspoon crushed red pepper, optional

Shake all the ingredients together in a jar with a tight-fitting lid. Store for up to 6 months.

> **Tip:** Mix into Cashew Sour Cream (page 236) for a quick dip.

HARISSA

MAKES: ½ cup (50 g) // **TIME:** 5 minutes

This spice blend is inspired by the North African and Middle Eastern chile paste. It really shines in dishes with tomato paste, onions, and olive oil. The combination may sound odd, but it really works. Bonus: This blend is surprisingly good for digestion, as cumin, caraway, and mint all help to eliminate gas and bloating. Stir this into Cashew Cream (page 236), squeeze in plenty of lemon juice, then use as a creamy spiced dip for toasted pita.

Grind the caraway, coriander, and cumin in a clean coffee grinder. Transfer to a jar with a tight-fitting lid; add the mint, garlic powder, paprika, and crushed red pepper, if using; and shake until combined. Store for up to 6 months.

2 tablespoons caraway seeds

2 tablespoons coriander seeds

2 tablespoons cumin seeds

2 teaspoons dried mint

2 teaspoons garlic powder

1 teaspoon sweet paprika

1 teaspoon crushed red pepper, optional

Tip: The capsaicin that gives chile peppers their spicy punch is also responsible for their anti-inflammatory properties. And once the heat from chiles subsides, you get an endorphin release, much like a runner's high after a tough workout! Chiles have also been found to improve heart health, alleviate congestion, and improve blood glucose levels.

SPRING ALL-PURPOSE SEASONING

SERVINGS: ½ cup (50 g) // **TIME:** 5 minutes

We think this trio of spring herbs is highly underrated. Pair this seasoning blend with fresh spring greens, braised white beans, and anything with lemon. Tarragon may not be used frequently here in the States, but it is a common addition in French cooking. It adds a fresh, sweet, subtle licorice flavor.

3 tablespoons dried dill

3 tablespoons dried thyme

2 tablespoons dried tarragon

Shake all the ingredients together in a jar with a tight-fitting lid. Store for up to 6 months.

FALL & WINTER
ALL-PURPOSE SEASONING

MAKES: about ½ cup (50 g) // **TIME:** 5 minutes

We're big fans of eating seasonally, so our go-to herb blends shift with the time of year. In winter, we season beans and roasted veggies with this hearty blend. Rosemary, thyme, and sage all provide protection for the respiratory and immune systems—a good reason to reach for them in colder months.

Use a mortar and pestle or coffee grinder to roughly grind the rosemary and sage. Transfer to a jar with a tight-fitting lid; add the thyme, pepper, and ginger, if using; and shake until combined. Store for up to 6 months.

3 tablespoons dried rosemary

2 tablespoons plus 2 teaspoons dried sage

2 tablespoons plus 2 teaspoons dried thyme

1 teaspoon black pepper

¼ teaspoon ground ginger, optional

KOREAN TAHINI BBQ SAUCE

MAKES: about ¾ cup (180 ml) sauce, 1¼ cup (300 ml) marinade // **TIME:** 10 minutes

Korean BBQ sauce is tangy, sweet, and spicy like its American counterpart, but with slightly more exotic ingredients and flavors. This simple sauce is surprisingly versatile, and it can be kid-friendly if you scale back the chili paste.

½ cup (120 ml) water

¼ cup (60 g) red miso

1-inch (2.5 cm) piece ginger, peeled and minced

3 cloves garlic, minced

2 tablespoons chili paste or chili sauce

2 tablespoons rice vinegar

2 tablespoons tahini

1 tablespoon dark brown sugar

½ teaspoon crushed red pepper, optional

Puree all the ingredients in a mini blender until smooth. Serve as is or thin with an additional ½ cup (120 ml) water and use as a marinade for tofu, tempeh, or portobello mushroom caps.

OF GFO FF

MISO GRAVY

SERVES: 8 to 12 / Makes about 3 cups (720 ml) // **TIME:** 15 minutes

The Naam in Vancouver boasts a spectacular beet burger served with sesame-turmeric oven fries (try our version on page 173!) and a rich yet balanced miso sauce we just had to replicate. We were pleasantly surprised to find that this sauce works best when it's completely oil-free! It has more of a kick than traditional gravy, but you can scale down the sweetness and intensity by using half the maple syrup and nutritional yeast.

1 Place a medium saucepan over medium heat. Add the flour and garlic. Cook, stirring often, until the garlic is soft and the flour smells toasty, about 3 minutes.

2 Increase the heat to medium-high and add the water, whisking constantly. When the mixture starts to thicken, remove from the heat. (This should take about 3 minutes, and it will be pourable but require the assistance of a spatula.)

3 Use a spatula to transfer the garlic-flour mixture to a blender; add the nutritional yeast, miso, vinegar, maple syrup, tahini, and pepper. Starting on low and working up to high, blend until thoroughly combined.

4 Taste and adjust seasoning as needed, and serve. (The gravy can be refrigerated in an airtight container for up to 4 days.)

½ cup (75 g) whole wheat flour (GF: ½ cup/50 g GF oats)

2 garlic cloves, chopped

2½ cups (600 ml) water

½ cup (15 g) nutritional yeast

3 tablespoons red miso

2 tablespoons apple cider vinegar

2 tablespoons maple syrup

2 tablespoons tahini

¼ teaspoon black pepper

Salt to taste

B-SAVORY SAUCE & MARINADE

MAKES: about 1¼ cups (360 ml) // **TIME:** 10 minutes

This umami-packed sauce is so-named because it's also packed with B vitamins, thanks to the nutritional yeast. We add turmeric and black pepper, which complement each other both nutrition-ally and in taste, plus balsamic and cider vinegars and vegan Worcestershire for richness and depth. The result is an intensely flavored oil-free sauce that can be added to almost any savory dish: Try it in stocks, soups, and stews; on cooked vegetables, grains, and legumes; and as a marinade for tem-peh, tofu, and mushrooms. Traditional Worcestershire is made with anchovies, so look for brands such as Annie's or Edward & Sons that have "vegan" on the label. And use a good balsamic, one that's rich and syrupy, like the Napa Valley Naturals brand.

½ cup (15 g) nutritional yeast

¼ cup (60 ml) reduced-sodium, GF tamari

2 tablespoons apple cider vinegar

2 tablespoons balsamic vinegar

2 tablespoons GF Worcestershire sauce

1 tablespoon plus 1 teaspoon maple syrup

2 teaspoons GF Dijon mustard

½ teaspoon ground turmeric

¼ teaspoon black pepper

Combine all the ingredients in a resealable container. The sauce can be refrigerated for up to 3 weeks, and it yields enough to marinate 4 blocks of tempeh or tofu, or 16 portobello caps.

VEGAN BASIL PESTO

SERVES: 4 to 6 / Makes 1 heaping cup (250 ml) // **TIME:** 5 minutes

Pesto is such an easy flavor boost for everything from steamed greens and baked potatoes to tofu sandwiches and guacamole (try it!). Though basil is the base of the classic pesto Genovese, you can swap in any herb or green for an interesting twist. The trick to retaining depth of flavor after ditching umami-laden Parmesan is the specific mix of nuts.

1 Pulse the basil, spinach, almonds, pine nuts, Brazil nuts, and garlic in a food processor until combined and finely chopped. With the food processor running, stream in the oil, stopping when it reaches the desired consistency. Add ¼ teaspoon salt, then added more to taste if desired.

2 The pesto can be refrigerated in an airtight container for up to 5 days. (OF: The oil helps preserve the pesto, so you'll want to use this within 1 day or freeze it.) It can also be frozen in single portions for up to 6 months: Scoop into ice cube trays, freeze, then transfer to an airtight container.

NOTE: *Basil tends to brown after being cut. The spinach keeps the pesto bright green.*

Variation: For Pesto Vinaigrette, whisk ¼ cup (60 ml) red wine vinegar into 2 tablespoons pesto.

2 bunches basil, leaves only

1 cup (40 g) spinach (see Note)

¼ cup (30 g) roasted almonds

¼ cup (30 g) toasted pine nuts

4 raw Brazil nuts, chopped

2 garlic cloves

¼ cup (60 ml) olive oil
(OF: ¼ cup/60 ml water)

¼ to ½ teaspoon salt

CHIMICHURRI

SERVES: 4 to 6 / Makes about 1 cup (240 ml) // **TIME:** 5 minutes

This thick herb sauce was inspired by a vegetarian restaurant in Barcelona called, simply, "Organic." In summer, you can drizzle it over grilled vegetables or use in place of pesto. It's also delightful swirled into hummus. Since the Argentines traditionally serve this on grilled meat, we suggest pairing it with mushrooms.

1 cup (15 g) flat-leaf parsley leaves

Grated zest and juice of 2 lemons

4 garlic cloves

1 teaspoon dried oregano

¼ cup (60 ml) olive oil (OF: water)

❶ Pulse the parsley, lemon zest and juice, garlic, and oregano in a food processor until combined. With the food processor running, stream in the oil, stopping when it reaches the desired consistency.

❷ The chimichurri can be refrigerated in an airtight container for up to 5 days. (OF: The oil helps preserve the chimichurri, so you'll want to use this within 1 day.) It can also be frozen in single portions for up to 6 months: Scoop into ice cube trays, freeze, then transfer to an airtight container.

Variation: Swap in nutritious greens such as nettles or dandelion.

CILANTRO-COCONUT PESTO

SERVES: 6 to 8 / Makes about 2 cups (480 ml) // **TIME:** 5 minutes

Taking its inspiration from Southeast Asia, this pesto adds flair to cooked grains, spices up sweet potatoes, and can be the base for a quick ramen noodle dish when simmered with vegetable broth. Toss with rice noodles, shredded carrots, and crunchy mung bean sprouts.

Process the coconut milk, cilantro, jalapeños, ginger, and miso in a blender until smooth. Thin with water as needed. The pesto can be refrigerated for up to 2 days, or divided into resealable containers and frozen for up to 6 months.

One 13.5-ounce (400 ml) can full-fat coconut milk

1 bunch cilantro, leaves only

2 jalapeños (seeds and ribs removed for less heat)

1-inch (2.5 cm) piece ginger, peeled and minced

1 tablespoon white miso

Water, as needed

CASHEW CREAM

SERVES: 4 to 6 / Makes about 2 cups (320 g) // **TIME:** 10 minutes, plus 1 hour to soak cashews

Rich yet simple, cashew cream is used in recipes throughout this book as a replacement for dairy. Cashew cream is not our creation; it's a staple of vegan comfort cuisine—and a revelation for anyone who thinks they could never go vegan because they can't give up dairy. Use a dollop anywhere you need to add some richness. We also share some quick variations that can stand in for other dairy ingredients. If your blender has a tamper, use that to help get a smooth texture without adding more water. Cashew cream should have the consistency of sour cream, but it will not have much tang.

1 cup (120 g) raw cashews, soaked in hot water for 1 hour, then drained

1 teaspoon fresh lemon juice

½ teaspoon salt

½ to 1 cup (120 to 240 ml) water

Combine the cashews, lemon juice, and salt in a high-speed blender, using a tamper to assist with blending. Add water 2 tablespoons at a time as needed to achieve desired consistency, and process until thick and creamy. (We typically need 1 cup/240 ml water, but start with ½ cup/120 ml.)

FF: *Make a batch every week and stash in the fridge so it will be on hand when you need it. (You'll always need it!) You can also scoop it into an ice cube tray and freeze, then transfer to a sealed container for up to 3 months. A single cube (just shy of 2 tablespoons) adds a hint of creaminess to oil-free dishes and simple soups that need a little something extra.*

CASHEW SOUR CREAM

Mix 1 cup (160 g) cashew cream with 2 teaspoons apple cider vinegar and 2 teaspoons fresh lemon juice. Season with salt as needed. Makes about 1 cup (160 g).

LIGHT CASHEW CREAM

Whisk ½ cup (120 ml) vegetable broth or water with 1 cup (160 g) cashew cream. This should have the consistency of actual cream. Makes 1½ cups (360 ml).

CASHEW MILK

Puree 1 cup (120 g) raw cashews with 1 cup (240 ml) water until smooth. This is deliberately unsweetened and plain, for use in savory dishes. Makes about 2 cups (480 ml).

CASHEW CREAM CHEESE

Add ¼ cup (15 g) nutritional yeast and ¼ teaspoon onion powder to the blender with the other ingredients. This should be thick and spreadable. Makes 2¼ cups (320 g).

Variation: For a "garden" cream cheese, stir in 1 scallion (white and light green parts), sliced; ¼ red bell pepper, minced; and 1 small grated carrot.

CASHEW QUESO

SERVES: 6 to 8 / Makes about 2 cups (320 g) // **TIME:** 15 minutes

A couple of years back, Stepf brought a huge bowl of this queso dip to a party hosted by *No Meat Athlete* editor Doug Hay and his wife, Katie. We all kept sneaking over to the bowl for more; it was just *so* good. Turns out, she had thrown it together earlier in the day as an experiment. Sometimes we PR without even trying; this was one of those times. Toss with quinoa and a green veggie for a cleaner spin on mac and cheese.

1 Process the cashews, nutritional yeast, garlic, chipotle, arrow-root powder, paprika, and water in a high-speed blender until it is thick yet pourable.

2 Transfer to a medium saucepan and heat over medium until bubbly, adding additional water if necessary. Season with salt and serve. (The queso will thicken as it cools, but whisking in some water can help loosen it up.)

3 Store in an airtight container in the refrigerator for up to 5 days.

Variation: For a milder Roasted Red Pepper Queso, substitute 1 roasted red bell pepper for the chipotle.

1 cup (120 g) raw cashews, soaked in hot water for at least 10 minutes, then drained

¼ cup (15 g) nutritional yeast

1 garlic clove

1 GF chipotle chile in adobo sauce (OF: 1 teaspoon chipotle chile powder or to taste)

1 teaspoon arrowroot powder

¼ teaspoon smoked paprika

¾ cup (180 ml) water, plus more as needed

Salt

MARINATED TOFU FETA

SERVES: 4 to 6 / Makes 1 pound (454 g) // **TIME:** 5 minutes to prep, plus 1 hour to marinate

This recipe turns firm tofu into a wonderful stand-in for marinated feta atop Greek salads. You can even skip the oil and you'll never notice. The first time we served this, everyone was sneaking bites out of the bowl while dinner cooked. That doesn't often happen with uncooked tofu!

2 tablespoons fresh lemon juice

½ teaspoon dried oregano

½ teaspoon salt

⅛ teaspoon crushed red pepper

⅛ teaspoon garlic powder

One 16-ounce (454 g) package sprouted or extra-firm tofu, drained and crumbled

1 tablespoon olive oil (OF: omit)

Combine the lemon juice, oregano, salt, crushed red pepper, and garlic powder in a large glass container with a lid. Add the tofu and toss to combine. Add the oil and toss again. Refrigerate for at least 1 hour or up to 3 days before serving.

Variation: This same seasoning blend is also great with artichokes. Drain and rinse 1 can of artichokes packed in water, place in a glass container with a lid, add the marinade, and cover with water. Or pour this right on top of frozen artichokes. Marinate for 1 day, tossing occasionally, for best results.

CASHEW TZATZIKI

SERVES: 4 to 6 / Makes ¾ cup (95 g) // **TIME:** 10 minutes, not including time to make Cashew Cream

This condiment is perfect for dressing up simple Mediterranean food, from falafel to Greek Chopped Salad (page 139). Sometimes we serve this creamy cucumber sauce with Indian food and call it *raita*, adding a ¼ teaspoon each of cumin seeds and ground cumin for smokiness. It's also a great topping for Olive-Chickpea Waffles (page 178).

Combine all the ingredients in a medium bowl. Serve immediately or refrigerate in an airtight container for up to 2 days.

NOTE: *The lemon juice and cucumber juices should loosen up the Cashew Cream, but if it's too thick for your liking, add water 1 tablespoon at a time.*

½ cup (50 g) chopped English cucumber

¼ cup (40 g) Cashew Cream (page 236)

1 teaspoon fresh lemon juice

¼ teaspoon garlic powder

⅛ teaspoon black pepper

QUICK PICKLED ONIONS

SERVES: 18 to 24 / Makes about 2½ cups (390 g) // **TIME:** 5 minutes to prep, plus 30 minutes to marinate

These onions (which aren't technically pickled, we know) add a little something special to everything from sandwiches and wraps to hummus and salsa. A pair of recipes from vegan cooking goddess Terry Hope Romero inspired this version, and "pickled" onions quickly became one of Matt's kids' favorite condiments (see Note). Add to Latin dishes, Indian dishes, salads, and anything else that needs a little extra zing.

2 large red onions, sliced in half and halves sliced thin

¼ cup (60 ml) fresh lime juice or lemon juice (from 2 limes or lemons)

1 tablespoon apple cider vinegar

2 teaspoons salt

¼ teaspoon sugar

1 Bring a large pot of water to a boil. Place the onions in a strainer set in the sink and pour the boiling water over the onions. After a few seconds, rinse under cold water.

2 Stir the lime juice, vinegar, salt, and sugar together in a large bowl, then add the onions. Cover and refrigerate for at least 30 minutes before using. (The pickled onions can be refrigerated for up to 6 weeks.)

NOTE: *For onions that have a milder, kid-friendly flavor with less bite, boil the onions for 30 seconds or so, then drain and rinse under cold water.*

SPICY PICKLED CARROTS

SERVES: 18 to 24 / Makes 3 cups (330 g) // **TIME:** 10 minutes, plus 8 to 24 hours to marinate

These carrots are a quick-fix version of those little jars of deliciousness you see at authentic taco trucks. Prep them the night before for maximum spiciness. Try them in taco salads or a Lifesaving Bowl (page 88).

Combine the carrots, vinegar, jalapeño, sugar, cumin, and salt in a quart-size (1 L) canning jar. Press the carrots down and add water just to cover. Put the lid on and shake to combine. Refrigerate 8 hours or overnight, then serve. (The carrots can be refrigerated for up to 1 week—though they likely won't last that long!)

4 carrots, grated

¼ cup (60 ml) apple cider vinegar

1 jalapeño, thinly sliced (seeds and ribs removed for less heat)

1 teaspoon sugar

½ teaspoon cumin seeds

½ teaspoon salt

Water

MINIMALIST GUACAMOLE

SERVES: 1 to 2 / Makes about 1 cup (240 g) // **TIME:** 5 minutes

There's real guacamole and then there's the quick stuff we make for avocado toast and topping salads and our Lifesaving Bowl (page 88). This minimalist version is kept simple because it's designed to blend in rather than be the star of a meal. See the Avocado Toast variations on page 58 for add-in ideas to really rock your guac.

1 avocado, mashed

2 tablespoons fresh lime juice

1 scallion (white and light green parts), sliced thin

Crushed red pepper

Salt

Combine the avocado, lime juice, and scallion in a small bowl. Season with crushed red pepper and salt and serve.

CHIPOTLE-PUMPKIN SEED SALSA

SERVES: 8 to 12 / Makes about 4 cups (985 g) // **TIME:** 15 minutes

Chips and salsa are a popular snack, but it's so easy to plow through those tiny store-bought jars of salsa—so we make our own when time allows. In this recipe, the pumpkin seeds thicken the salsa and add texture and nutrition (fiber, protein, iron, and zinc). Use the higher amount of chipotles if you prefer more smokiness and heat.

1 Place a medium skillet over low heat and add the pumpkin seeds. Toast, stirring often, until fragrant and light brown, about 3 minutes. Transfer to a medium bowl and set aside.

2 Increase the heat to medium-high, then add the onion and garlic. (Add a splash of water if the pan looks dry or garlic begins to brown.) Cook, stirring occasionally to avoid burning, about 3 minutes. Stir in the chipotle(s) and cook for 1 minute. Stir in the tomatoes with their juice and cook, without stirring, for 5 minutes. Remove from the heat and stir again.

3 While the tomato mixture is cooking, transfer the pumpkin seeds to a food processor. Pulse several times, until the seeds are partially ground with some larger pieces. Return the seeds to the bowl.

4 Add the tomato mixture to the now-empty food processor. Pulse several times, add ¼ teaspoon salt, and pulse until the salsa is uniform in texture.

5 Transfer to the bowl with the pumpkin seeds, stir to combine, and season with salt. Serve or refrigerate in an airtight container for up to 3 days.

½ cup (80 g) raw pumpkin seeds

1 yellow onion, diced

3 garlic cloves, minced

1 or 2 GF chipotles chiles in adobo sauce, chopped (OF: 1 or 2 teaspoons chipotle chile powder or to taste)

One 28-ounce (794 g) can diced tomatoes with juice

¼ teaspoon salt, plus more to taste

PINEAPPLE SALSA

SERVES: 6 to 8 / Makes about 3 cups (630 g) // **TIME:** 10 minutes

This salsa is courtesy of a food-critic friend, Polly, known for her simple yet memorable food. The pineapple is refreshing and somewhat unexpected, making this just different enough to seem impressive, yet it takes almost no time to prepare. Serve it with Slow-Cooker Refried Beans (page 174) and brown rice for a quick supper.

1 pound (455 g) fresh or thawed frozen pineapple, finely diced, juices reserved

1 white or red onion, finely diced

1 bunch cilantro or mint, leaves only, chopped

1 jalapeño, minced, optional

Salt

Combine the pineapple with its juice, onion, cilantro, and jalapeño, if using, in a medium bowl. Season with salt to taste and serve. (For even more flavor, refrigerate overnight before serving. The salsa can be refrigerated in an airtight container for up to 2 days.)

BEER "CHEESE" DIP

SERVES: 8 to 12 / Makes about 3 cups (720 ml) // **TIME:** 15 minutes, not including time to soak nuts

This tangy, versatile dip is inspired by *The Full Helping* blog's vegan walnut-cheddar recipe. If you miss fondue, try this with toasted chunks of soft pretzel, apple slices, and blanched broccoli. Or pour it over a baked potato and top with loads of scallions. You can even use it as pasta sauce. Serve with more beer, if you must. (We told you it was versatile.)

1 Puree the beer, water, cashews, walnuts, lemon juice, tomato paste, and vinegar in a high-speed blender until completely smooth.

2 Transfer to a medium saucepan set over medium heat. Whisk in the nutritional yeast, arrowroot powder, and paprika. Cook, whisking often, until the mixture thickens, about 7 minutes. Remove from the heat, whisk in the miso paste, and serve immediately.

3 Store in an airtight container in the refrigerator for up to 5 days.

NOTE: *For a "sharp" cheddar taste, use tomato paste. For a mild flavor, use the roasted red pepper.*

¾ cup (180 ml) brown ale

¾ cup (180 ml) water

½ cup (60 g) raw cashews, soaked in hot water for at least 15 minutes, then drained

½ cup (60 g) raw walnuts, soaked in hot water for at least 15 minutes, then drained

2 tablespoons fresh lemon juice

2 tablespoons tomato paste or 1 roasted red pepper

1 tablespoon apple cider vinegar

½ cup (30 g) nutritional yeast

1 tablespoon arrowroot powder

½ teaspoon sweet or smoked paprika

1 tablespoon red miso

SPANISH RED PEPPER SPREAD (ROMESCO)

SERVES: 8 to 12 / Makes about 2 cups (595 g) // **TIME:** 15 minutes

This classic Spanish dip feels fancy but comes together quickly. It's sweet and smoky, and slightly crunchy yet creamy. We love to dollop it on cooked grains or steamed vegetables, spread it on a veggie sandwich or toast, or use it as a vegetable dip.

½ cup (60 g) raw almonds or walnuts

1 slice whole wheat bread, chopped

2 garlic cloves

One 15-ounce (425 g) jar roasted red peppers, drained (with liquid reserved) and rinsed

3 tablespoons chopped flat-leaf parsley

¼ cup (60 ml) olive oil (OF: ¼ cup/65 g pureed white beans)

1 Toast the almonds in a small skillet over medium heat for about 3 minutes, shaking occasionally, until golden brown and fragrant. Remove from the heat and transfer to a food processor.

2 Add the bread and garlic to the now-empty skillet. Cook until the bread is toasted and the garlic is soft, about 3 minutes.

3 Transfer to the food processor with the almonds and pulse a few times. Add the red peppers and parsley and pulse until well blended, then drizzle in the olive oil and liquid from the red pepper jar until the dip is uniform in texture but quite thick. Serve.

4 Store in an airtight container in the refrigerator for up to 5 days.

EMERGENCY VEGAN SHAKIN' BITS

SERVES: 6 to 8 / Makes about 1¾ cups (225 g) // **TIME:** 10 minutes

As athletes fueled by plants, we're accustomed to planning ahead, being creative, and making special requests when dining out. Still, how many times have you been promised a "chef's special," only to be served a plate of steamed veggies? We've been there. Keep a small shaker bottle of this savory topping in your bag when you travel. Discreetly bring it out and shake it over those dull veggies or plain rice for a big boost of flavor (not to mention protein, healthy fats, fiber, and micronutrients).

Pulse all the ingredients in a spice grinder until thoroughly combined. Store in an airtight container for up to 3 months.

½ cup (80 g) hemp seeds

½ cup (75 g) raw sunflower seeds

¼ cup (40 g) flaxseeds

¼ cup (15 g) nutritional yeast

¼ cup (40 g) raw pumpkin seeds

¼ cup (7 g) dried wakame, optional

1 ounce (30 g) dried mushrooms, crumbled

1 teaspoon black pepper

½ teaspoon garlic powder

½ teaspoon ground turmeric

¼ teaspoon salt, optional

Chapter 9

DOUBLE-DUTY DESSERTS: SWEETS THAT WORK FOR YOUR BODY

Who says dessert is a forbidden indulgence during training? Sweet treats like Pineapple Soft-Serve, Two-Ingredient Peanut Butter Fudge, and Banana Cream Chia Pudding Parfaits are packed with ingredients that actually support your healthy lifestyle.

Of course, we also have recipes for a few desserts that are a bit more decadent, such as Triple Chocolate Icebox Cake, No-Bake Mocha Cheesecake, and Black Sesame–Ginger Quick Bread. Because every now and then, we like a little indulgence, too. And fortunately, if you limit foods with added sugars, refined carbohydrates, and oils to less than 10 percent of your total calories, it's likely that your body won't really notice a difference. Just don't let 10 percent become 20; for some people it's a very slippery slope.

One particularly great thing about vegan desserts: We've noticed they're an ideal introduction to a plant-based diet for family and friends. You might think that without eggs and butter, vegan desserts wouldn't stand a chance at a potluck full of omnivores, but we hear more "I could be vegan if I had you to cook for me!" comments about desserts than any other dish. And once you have them convinced that vegan desserts can hold their own against more traditional ones, you might even persuade them to try some savory dishes next! OK, so they may not be running home to throw away all the animal products in their house, but it's a start; we like to spread our message in a way that's convincing without being pushy, and sharing food that everyone loves is one of the best ways to do it.

BASIC VANILLA CHIA PUDDING

SERVES: 2 to 4 // **TIME:** 20 minutes

While some people consider chia pudding to be a breakfast dish, this one definitely falls into the dessert category. We use dark sugar for a rich sweetness, plus a mix of almond and coconut milks for a more dessert-like flavor. If you do prefer to eat this for breakfast, you can make it lighter by using all almond milk instead of adding coconut milk.

Whisk all the ingredients together in a medium bowl. Stir every few minutes until thickened, about 15 minutes. Serve, or refrigerate for up to 48 hours. If necessary, whisk in a bit of water before serving.

NOTE: *Use vanilla bean paste or powder rather than extract in dishes that won't be cooked. Vanilla extract can have a harsh, alcoholic flavor in recipes that aren't heated.*

1 cup (240 ml) almond milk

½ cup (120 ml) full-fat coconut milk

⅓ cup (65 g) chia seeds

1 tablespoon dark sugar (raw sugar, dark brown sugar, or coconut sugar), or to taste

1 teaspoon vanilla bean powder (see Note)

Pinch of salt

BANANA CREAM CHIA PUDDING PARFAITS

MAKES: 2 parfaits // **TIME:** 20 minutes, not including time to make Basic Vanilla Chia Pudding

These parfaits were inspired by banoffee pie, which is a delightful combination of banana and caramel. We've swapped in nature's caramel (aka dates) along with chia pudding for a nutrient-packed sweet treat.

½ batch Basic Vanilla Chia Pudding (page 249)

1 banana, sliced

4 dates, pitted and chopped fine

4 vegan gingersnaps or vanilla cookies

Layer all the ingredients in the order listed, dividing them evenly between two glasses. Serve right away or refrigerate overnight, which will allow time for the cookies to soften.

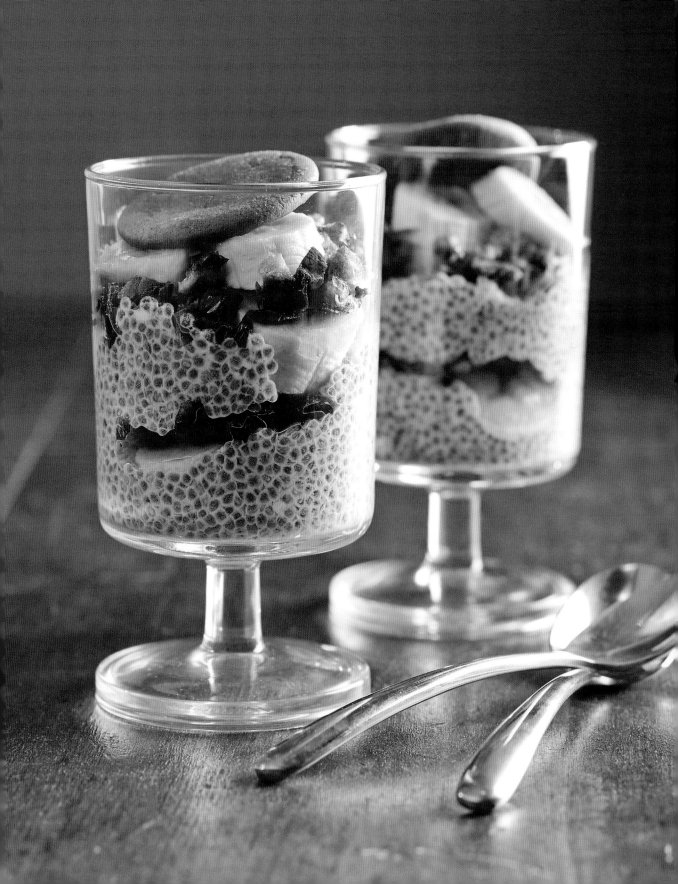

MANGO STICKY RICE

SERVES: 4 to 6 // **TIME:** 45 minutes

When you are carbo-loading, this is the perfect whole food dessert. We sweeten short-grain brown rice with coconut milk and dark brown sugar, then add lime juice and top with mango. The only "trick" is that your mango needs to be really ripe and sweet. That's it! No fresh mango? Swap in whatever's in season: peaches, berries, or even ripe pears.

2½ cups (600 ml) water

1 cup (180 g) short-grain brown rice

½ cup (120 ml) light or full-fat coconut milk

2 tablespoons dark brown sugar or coconut sugar

1 to 2 tablespoons fresh lime juice, to taste

2 mangos, peeled and diced

Unsweetened shredded coconut, optional

1 Bring the water to a boil in a medium saucepan, then lower the heat to medium-low and stir in the rice. Cook, stirring often, until the liquid is absorbed and the rice is tender, about 30 minutes.

2 Remove from the heat and stir in the coconut milk and sugar. Add lime juice to taste, then pour into a shallow glass dish. Top with mango, garnish with coconut, if desired, and serve. (This dish can also be refrigerated and served cold, but wait to garnish with the coconut until just before serving.)

SWEET RED BEANS

SERVES: 4 to 6 // **TIME:** 30 to 45 minutes, not including time to soak beans

In Japan, China, and Korea, small red beans are sweetened and served as dessert. Trust us on this one: Cooked with vanilla and maple syrup, they have a satisfying texture and a rich, chocolate-like flavor. Adzuki beans are rich in antioxidants, fiber, and all the other goodness beans provide. Serve them warm as a protein-packed topping for ice cream or oatmeal, or spread them on pancakes, waffles, or cinnamon-raisin toast. Be sure to also try them on top of a Frozen Matcha Latte (page 199) for an almost-authentic Asian treat.

1 Place the beans and vanilla in a medium saucepan. Add the water and bring to a boil. Cover and continue to boil until tender, about 30 minutes. (If your beans are still tough and need more water to cook, add it sparingly; you don't want soupy beans.)

2 Remove from the heat and stir in the sugar and salt. Let cool before serving.

1 cup (205 g) adzuki beans, soaked overnight, drained and rinsed

¼ teaspoon vanilla bean powder or ½ teaspoon vanilla extract

2 cups (360 ml) water

3 tablespoons raw sugar or maple syrup, or more to taste

⅛ teaspoon salt

PINEAPPLE SOFT-SERVE

SERVES: 2 // **TIME:** 5 minutes

This fluffy pineapple soft-serve is inspired by the trademarked version served at Disney parks. Ours has just two ingredients with no added sugar. (For a dessert that's closer to the original, add 1 tablespoon raw sugar.) You can turn just about any fruit into dessert, as long as you have a blender that's up to the task.

One 10-ounce (284 g) bag frozen pineapple

2 tablespoons to ¼ cup (60 ml) vanilla almond milk

Process the pineapple in a high-speed blender on high while tamping down for 30 seconds. Add the almond milk as needed while processing and tamping for another 30 seconds, until silky smooth. Serve immediately.

Variations:

Blueberry-Lime-Coconut: Use one 12-ounce (340 g) bag frozen blueberries, zest and juice of 1 lime, and up to ½ cup (120 ml) light or full-fat coconut milk.

Strawberry-Banana: Use one 12-ounce (340 g) bag frozen strawberries plus 1 frozen banana, with up to ½ cup (120 ml) vanilla almond milk.

Mango: Use one 12-ounce (340 g) bag frozen mango, zest and juice of 1 lime, and up to ½ cup (120 ml) light or full-fat coconut milk.

Raspberry-Orange: Use one 12-ounce (340 g) bag frozen raspberries, zest and juice of 1 orange, and up to ¼ cup (60 ml) light or full-fat coconut milk.

TWO-INGREDIENT PEANUT BUTTER FUDGE

SERVES: 6 to 8 // **TIME:** 5 minutes

Making candy the traditional way sounds a little scary: thermometers and boiling hot sugar? No, thanks. This two-ingredient version yields the same creamy texture without the fear of dripping molten sugar onto yourself. The fudge freezes well, too. Feel free to swap in another nut butter for the peanut butter.

1 cup (160 g) chocolate chips

½ cup (130 g) natural peanut butter

Sea salt

1 Place the chocolate chips and peanut butter in a small saucepan over medium-low heat. Cook, stirring often, until the chocolate is melted and the mixture is thoroughly combined, about 5 minutes. Use a spatula to scrape the mixture into a pie plate or small glass container lined with parchment paper. Sprinkle with sea salt.

2 Refrigerate until set, at least 1 hour or overnight. Slice into squares and serve, or refrigerate for up to 1 week.

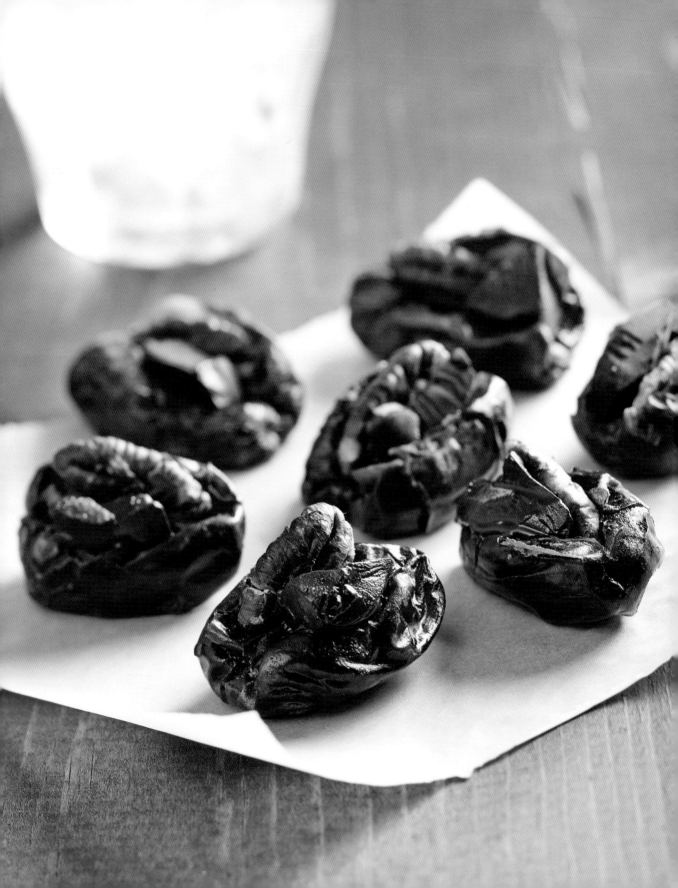

TWO-MINUTE TURTLES

MAKES: 12 turtles // **TIME:** 5 minutes

These are perfect for those times when you just need something small and sweet: You stuff two items inside a date, heat it, and eat it. They taste like candy, so you will feel as if you created something special each time you make them.

1 Slice lengthwise into each date, making sure to only go halfway through. Carefully widen the opening, then stuff in 1 pecan and a couple of chocolate chips.

2 Repeat with the remaining dates, pecans, and chocolate chips and serve. (Optional: Place the stuffed dates on a plate and microwave just until the chocolate is slightly warm, about 30 seconds. You can also warm them in a toaster oven set to low for about 5 minutes. Allow to cool slightly before serving.) The turtles can be stored in an airtight container for up to 2 days.

NOTE: *Chocolate chunks are easier to stuff into the dates, so use those if you have them at home.*

12 pitted dates

12 toasted pecans

¼ cup (40 g) chocolate chips

NO-BAKE MOCHA CHEESECAKE

MAKES: one 9-inch (23 cm) round cake // **TIME:** 50 minutes

No-bake vegan cheesecakes typically use a lot of coconut oil, and, as a result, they can feel heavy and coat the mouth. This version uses agar to aid the firming process instead of coconut oil. The result is a lighter yet still creamy mocha cake, definitely a special-occasion treat.

CRUST

12 chocolate sandwich cookies, such as Newman-O's (OF: 4 medium bananas, sliced)

FILLING

One 13.5-ounce (400 ml) can full-fat coconut milk

1 tablespoon agar flakes

1 tablespoon plus 1 teaspoon instant coffee

¼ cup (80 g) maple syrup

¼ cup (60 ml) water

½ teaspoon vanilla extract

1 cup (120 g) raw cashews, soaked in hot water for at least 10 minutes, then drained

2 tablespoons unsweetened cocoa powder

1 To make the crust, place the cookies in the bowl of a food processor. Pulse until roughly chopped, then process until they resemble crumbs. Pour into a 9-inch (23 cm) pie plate and press the crumbs to form a crust. Freeze it while you make the filling. (OF: Layer the sliced bananas in the bottom of the pie pan. Freezing is not necessary.)

2 To make the filling, transfer the solids from the coconut milk to a high-speed blender. Pour the liquid into a small saucepan. (Don't worry if some of the solids get in there. They'll melt.)

3 Add the agar, coffee, maple syrup, water, and vanilla to the saucepan with the liquids and whisk to combine. Place over medium heat and allow the mixture to come to a simmer, with tiny bubbles breaking the surface. Let cook for 3 minutes, whisking often, until the agar is completely dissolved.

4 Add the cashews and cocoa to the blender with the coconut milk solids. Process, pausing as needed to scrape down the sides, until smooth.

5 With the blender running on low, pour in the contents of the saucepan and process until the filling is smooth and thoroughly combined. Pour the filling into the prepared crust and refrigerate until set, at least 30 minutes. Serve chilled. (The cheesecake can be refrigerated for up to 5 days [OF: up to 2 days]. Individual slices can be frozen for up to 6 weeks.)

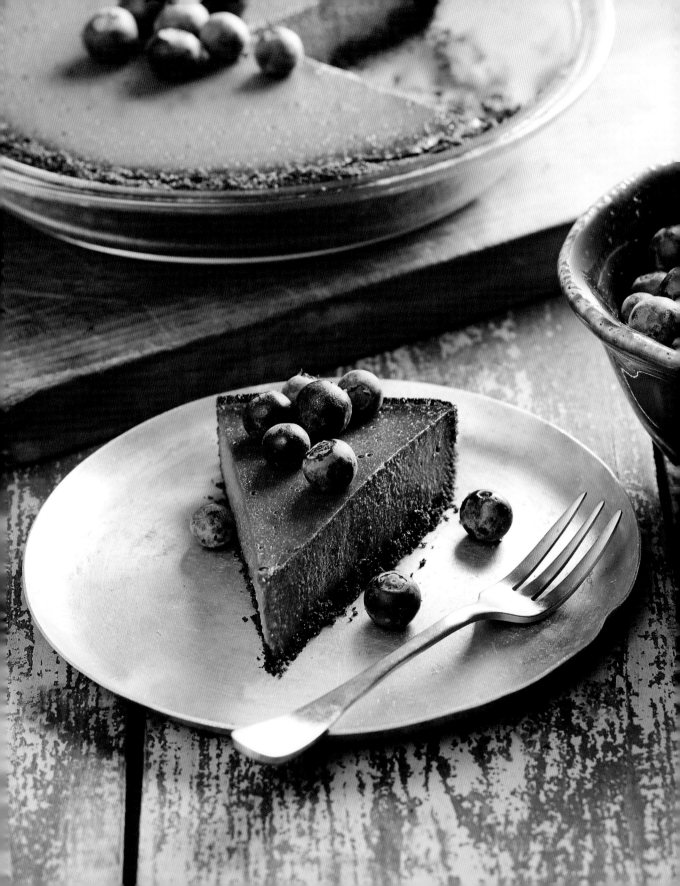

CHOCOLATE LAVA MUG CAKE

MAKES: 1 mug-size cake // **TIME:** 2 minutes, not including time to cook beans

Mug cakes are all the rage, and while a microwave is not one of our "must-have" kitchen items listed in Chapter 2, we do appreciate the ease it provides if you're cooking for one. This simple cake takes less than two minutes to cook and doesn't leave any leftovers. Plus, you don't have to share!

¼ cup (60 ml) almond milk

1 tablespoon cooked, unsweetened
   adzuki or black beans,
   mashed well

1 tablespoon sugar

½ teaspoon vanilla extract

2 tablespoons unsweetened
   cocoa powder

¼ cup (30 g) whole wheat
   pastry flour

⅛ teaspoon salt

¼ teaspoon baking powder

2 tablespoons mini chocolate chips

1 Combine the almond milk, beans, sugar, and vanilla in a mug. Stir in the cocoa, flour, salt, and baking powder until just combined. Drop the chocolate chips in the center.

2 Microwave until the cake is set around the edges but the center is soft, about 90 seconds. Let sit for 5 minutes, then eat!

NOTE: *Serve with drippy peanut or almond butter, if desired.*

TRIPLE CHOCOLATE ICEBOX CAKE

MAKES: one 9 x 5-inch (23 x 13 cm) cake // **TIME:** 20 minutes to prep, 1 hour to chill

Icebox cakes are one of the many things we discovered after moving to the South. The originals are definitely not vegan, so we plantified this classic summer dessert. It's fun to make and really good, too. If you want a bittersweet chocolate filling as a contrast to the sweet cookies, omit the maple syrup. Use any kind of sandwich cookie you like. This cake can be scaled down easily.

1 Combine the coconut milk, cocoa powder, and maple syrup, if using, in a blender until smooth.

2 Place a single layer of cookies in the bottom of a 9 x 5-inch (23 x 13 cm) loaf pan. (Use glass so you can see the layers.) Spread about a quarter of the filling on top. Repeat with the remaining cookies and filling. Cover and refrigerate for at least 1 hour or overnight.

3 To serve, use a butter knife to loosen the edges and invert onto a plate. (Or, simply scoop a serving into a bowl.) Sprinkle with mini chocolate chips, if using, before serving.

Variation: Omit the cocoa powder and substitute gingersnaps for the chocolate cookies.

One 13.5-ounce (400 ml) can light or full-fat coconut milk

¼ cup (20 g) unsweetened cocoa powder

2 tablespoons maple syrup, optional

One 13-ounce (368 g) package double chocolate sandwich cookies (we use Newman-O's) (OF: 4 medium bananas, sliced, and 1 cup/125 g raspberries)

2 tablespoons mini chocolate chips, optional

BLACK SESAME–GINGER QUICK BREAD

MAKES: 1 loaf or 12 muffins // **TIME:** 20 minutes to prep, 50 minutes to cook

This is a vegan version of a wonderful cake served at Dobra Tea in Asheville. The recipe might look finicky, but it's virtually foolproof. This hearty bread holds up just fine in a jersey pocket if wrapped in parchment paper.

⅔ cup (95 g) black sesame seeds

1 cup (65 g) candied ginger

1½ cups (180 g) plus 2 tablespoons whole wheat pastry flour

1 cup (110 g) almond meal

2½ teaspoons baking powder

½ teaspoon salt

¾ cup (180 ml) almond milk, room temperature

¾ cup (150 g) raw sugar

½ cup (120 ml) melted coconut oil (OF: ½ cup/120 g applesauce)

2 tablespoons chia seeds

1 tablespoon fresh lemon juice

1 tablespoon ginger juice (or 1 teaspoon ginger puree plus 2 teaspoons water)

1 Adjust an oven rack to the middle position, and preheat the oven to 350°F (180°C). Line a 9 x 5-inch (23 x 13 cm) loaf pan with parchment paper (or line two muffin pans with liners).

2 Pulse the sesame seeds in a food processor until ground. Transfer to a large bowl and set aside.

3 Add the ginger and 2 tablespoons of the flour to the food processor; pulse until the ginger is roughly chopped. (The flour will help keep it suspended in the batter as it bakes.)

4 Add the remaining flour, almond meal, baking powder, and salt to the bowl with the ground sesame seeds. Stir to combine, then stir in the ginger. Make a well in the center.

5 Process the almond milk, sugar, coconut oil, chia seeds, lemon juice, and ginger juice in the now-empty food processor until completely combined. Transfer to the bowl with the dry ingredients and gently fold in the wet ingredients until just combined. (The batter will be quite thick.)

6 Scoop the batter into the loaf pan. Smooth the top(s) with a wet spatula. Bake for 45 to 50 minutes (30 minutes for muffins), until a toothpick inserted in the center comes out clean.

7 Allow to cool for 10 minutes in the pan(s), then allow to cool completely on a rack before slicing or peeling off the liners.

Chapter 10

MEAL PLANNING:
MAKING THESE RECIPES WORK IN YOUR REAL LIFE

Astable of healthy, delicious meals is only half the battle; you also need a strategy for combining them day-to-day. This chapter ties together our nutrition philosophy and recipes with workable, adaptable meal plans to suit a variety of needs, plus guidelines for modifying or even constructing your own meal plan. We also offer several lists of recipes organized by training needs—whether you're looking to carbo-load, need a race-day or game-day breakfast, or are dreaming of a postrace feast—so that you can easily choose a recipe from the book to fit your situation. First up, let's see how you can fit these recipes—and cooking in general—into your training plan.

THE "DOUBLE-UP METHOD" OF WEEKLY MEAL PLANNING

Meal planning is immensely helpful when it comes to getting a healthy dinner on the table after a workout and a long day at the office or taking care of little ones. We know a lot of people shy away from this approach, thinking they need to cook an entire week's worth of food at once (though that's *an op-tion*, it's not the only one). But we also know that most people don't have time to whip up new recipes every night of the week (even if they are the simple ones from this book). Thankfully, there's a lot of middle ground between these two extremes.

With meal planning, a little goes a long way, and there are two approaches we recommend for beginners. One is to embrace the "cook once, eat twice" method of always cooking double the amount you'll need for one meal. It's straightforward and simple.

The other is what we like to call the "double-up method." During your busiest weeks, this method can mean the difference between healthy, home-cooked meals or takeout. The premise is simple: Pick two main dishes and cook them. (If you're feeding the whole family, you may need to make double batches of each.) You'll focus most of your creative cooking energy on those. Then, while you're at it, cook up two simple whole grains and two sauces, dressings, or condiments. By mixing and matching those two mains with the grains and sauces, you'll have plenty of options and avoid the boredom that comes with eating the same batch of curry or lentil soup for a week straight. Come mealtime, you'll only need to cook your vegetables, which you can also prep ahead of time.

To summarize, you'll make:

- 2 main dishes

- 2 simple whole grains

- 2 sauces, dressings, or condiments

To do this, set aside a couple of hours on a slow evening or your rest day. Do the usual meal prep: Take inventory of your kitchen, make a list, shop, prep, cook, and pack. Aside from replenishing greens (and perhaps vegetables) midweek, you should have your weeknight meals covered. (And, if you make enough food, your weekday lunches, too.)

TIP: *Save time by buying sauces and condiments with ingredient lists appropriate for your eating preferences.*

WHAT ABOUT VEGETABLES?

This part is the only real daily work. You should prep at least two vegetables, but feel free to overachieve here. Choose two different colors for each meal. One of your vegetables should be a dark leafy green.

RAW: Shredded carrots, beets, or red cabbage; chopped celery, broccoli, or cauliflower; diced cucumbers, red onion or scallions, or bell peppers (only prepare about two days' worth at a time); sprouts; pickled vegetables; etc.

COOKED: Roasted root vegetables, sautéed broccoli or cauliflower, leftover stir-fry veggies, etc.

GREENS: Kale, collards, chard, arugula, or mixed salad greens. Buy them whole and prep at home, or buy the big containers of mixed greens for convenience—they're triple-washed and ready to go. Choose what works for you. (In our experience, the baby greens tend to keep for a shorter time than hardier greens such as kale and arugula, so plan accordingly.)

A sample plan appears on the next page:

MAIN DISH	GRAIN	SAUCE
Slow-Cooker Refried Beans (page 174)	Quinoa	Lemon-Tahini Dressing (page 146)
Peanut Butter Tempeh (page 104)	Pearled Barley	Chipotle–Pumpkin Seed Salsa

assemble their own portion. You can reheat or eat straight from the fridge. You can add extra ingredients like fresh herbs, stuff it all into a burrito, or bake it into a casserole if you want. Even if you decide to get creative every night, you've already cut way down on the time it will take to get dinner into your face.

Prep the ingredients, label them, and store them in the fridge. When it's time to pack lunch or pull together dinner, grab what you want and pile it all in a bowl. You can serve family-style or each person can

If you're someone who likes to pack up and refrigerate a week's worth of food all at once, this is going to help you tremendously!

Here's how we put this plan into practice one week:

	MONDAY	TUESDAY	WEDNESDAY	THURSDAY	FRIDAY
LUNCH	Slow-Cooker Refried Beans (page 174) + quinoa + Lemon-Tahini Dressing (page 146) + baby kale + pickled vegetables	Slow-Cooker Refried Beans + barley + Chipotle–Pumpkin Seed Salsa (page 243) + avocado + spinach	Baked Tempeh Nuggets (page 170) + barley + Chipotle–Pumpkin Seed Salsa + spinach + shredded carrots	Baked Tempeh Nuggets + quinoa + Lemon-Tahini Dressing + baby kale + shredded carrots	Slow-Cooker Refried Beans + barley + Chipotle–Pumpkin Seed Salsa + frozen corn + baby kale
DINNER	Baked Tempeh Nuggets + barley + Chipotle–Pumpkin Seed Salsa + chopped bell peppers + spinach	Baked Tempeh Nuggets + quinoa + Lemon-Tahini Dressing + baby kale + roasted beets	Slow-Cooker Refried Beans + quinoa + Lemon-Tahini Dressing + arugula + frozen broccoli	Baked Tempeh Nuggets + barley + Chipotle–Pumpkin Seed Salsa + spinach (stuffed into whole wheat tortilla)	Slow-Cooker Refried Beans + quinoa + Lemon-Tahini Dressing + chopped tomatoes + spinach +Lemon-Tahini Dressing + chopped tomatoes + spinach

RECIPE LISTS

As athletes just like you, we know you will need specialized meals based on your training plan. We've created these lists to help support you throughout the year.

Carb-Loading Meals

Our meals provide plenty of the carbs you need to fuel your lengthier workouts, but the ones we've compiled here are some of our faves for those times you want to stockpile some energy reserves the day before a long workout or race.

RACE-DAY BREAKFASTS

Big-day jitters can be enough of a challenge for your GI system. Keep your stomach happy and fuel up for a PR with these morning meals.

Finish-Line Feasts

Does anyone else spend the hard miles dreaming of what you're going to eat after the race? We thought so. These finish-line feasts are worth the effort in the kitchen, if you have the energy left after giving your all on the trail. These meals are also really good for dinner parties, if your friends are into the same crazy feats you are.

PASTA PARTY

- Lemony Steamed Kale with Olives (page 161)
- Chocolate Lava Mug Cakes (page 260)

ITALIAN FEAST

- Simplified Spinach-Mushroom Lasagna (page 87)
- Roasted Garlic Dressing (page 148) with green salad
- No-Bake Mocha Cheesecake (page 258)

FINISH-LINE FIESTA

- Pinto Bean & Greens Enchilada Casserole (page 97)
- Creamy Avocado-Lime Dressing (page 151) with jicama, grapefruit, and arugula salad
- Pineapple–Black Bean Bowls with Roasted Veggies (page 96)

COMFORT FOOD BANQUET

- Peanut Butter Tempeh (page 104) with Miso Gravy (page 231)
- Smoky Potato Salad over Greens (page 143)

- Roasted Red Pepper Mac & Cheese (page 117)
- Triple Chocolate Icebox Cake (page 261)

ASIAN-INSPIRED

- Tahini Green Beans (page 158)
- Anti-Inflammatory Miso Soup (page 112)
- Black Sesame–Ginger Quick Bread (page 262)

CULINARY TOUR DE FRANCE

- French Onion Stew with Mushrooms (page 126)
- Provençal Potato Gratin (page 184)
- Classic French Vinaigrette (page 153) with mixed green salad

MEDITERRANEAN CRUISE

- Olive-Chickpea Waffles (page 178)
- Greek Chopped Salad (page 139)
- Olives & stuffed grape leaves (take help from the supermarket)

Acknowledgments

WE WOULD LIKE TO THANK:
Matthew, Jeanne, Joan, and the entire team at The Experiment for this opportunity.

Cindy Uh, for your support along the way.

Rich Roll, for your heartfelt contribution to our book and the generous, important work you do to bring attention to this plant-based movement and help create a more sustainable world.

Bren Dendy, for the beautiful photos in the book proposal.

Photographer Ken Carlson, art director Sarah Smith, and food stylist Sue Hoss for bringing our recipes to life.

Our devoted recipe testers: ultra-marathoner extraordinaire Amie Dworecki, poet Meghan Sterling, journalist and new mama Laura Arenschield (and Wes!), fledgling tofu entrepreneur Corrie Callaghan, the ever-calm and generous Sarah Carter, food stylist Lynne Morris, running coach Kristin Gordon-Hock, Sanctuary Brewing Company co-owner and vegan activist Lisa McDonald (and friends!), Dr. Shannon Ardaiolo, enthusiastic vegan cooks Kurt and Amanda Strecker (aka The Vegan Mama, whose son was just weeks old at the time!), BSM cycling wife Katie Lundbeck, cyclist and hiker Tiffany Royal, Gina Harney aka the Fitnessista, Stepf's BFF Misha Metcalf, and Coach Tony Viton, RD.

Sarah and Chad of Smiling Hara Tempeh for the tasty tempeh we used for recipe testing—and their commitment to sustainability and producing unique, delicious tempeh.

Miso Master (especially Marnie and Leila) for sharing your knowledge about this umami-rich ingredient, as well as the care packages of miso and sea veggies.

MATT WOULD LIKE TO THANK:
Stepfanie Romine, for drawing on your incredibly diverse culinary background to bring our shared vision for this book to life—healthily, practically, and deliciously.

Erin Frazier, for all the work you did to help us test these recipes, and for being the inspiration for everything I do. Holden Frazier, for being the only kid in Little League to have grape switchel in your water bottle, and loving it. Ellarie Frazier, for showing me what being a whole food eater really means.

Ray Cronise, for hours of thoughtful, mind-blowing conversation about nutrition and how to best convey this message we believe in, to give readers the best chance of transforming their health for the better.

Michael Greger and Joel Fuhrman, for the work you do to bring this whole food, plant-based message to the masses in a way that's trustworthy, engaging, and practical.

The No Meat Athlete team: Erin Frazier, Susan Lacke, Doug Hay, and Esther Brown. Without your dedication, loyalty, and unique gifts, No Meat Athlete wouldn't have touched a fraction of the lives we have.

Mom, Dad, and Christine Hein, for your endless support and encouragement, and helping me to see that this path (while not the default one) is the only one for me.

Members of the No Meat Athlete running groups around the world, and especially their leaders who have worked fearlessly and tirelessly to build groups in your cities that create friendships, support new plant-based athletes, and are a heck of a lot of fun.

Finally, the hundreds of thousands of No Meat Athlete readers and podcast listeners, each of whom changes the world just a little bit when you show up to the gym, to a race, or just to lunch as a proud, healthy plant-based athlete.

STEPFANIE WOULD LIKE TO THANK:

My coauthor, Matt Frazier, for the opportunity to work with you and the No Meat Athlete community. I have tremendous respect for you and the work you put in to provide fellow athletes with trustworthy, interesting content and education.

Sam Klontz, the world's greatest cat dad and husband, for taking care of so much while I wrote this book. I love you, and I couldn't have done this without you. I am especially grateful that you helped test recipes (and handled all the dishes and the grocery shopping)!

My sisters and dearest friends, Rachael DiFransico and Kaitlynn Fisher, whose texts are the best reality checks.

My Gaia Herbs family, for all the support and encouragement, and a special thanks to Beth, Ariel, Alison, Jenna, Tracey, Nichole, and Kristen.

Dr. Mary Bove, ND, for the herbal and holistic health education and inspiration you've given me. I'm forever grateful.

Jennifer Partlow, my loyal running partner, who's always right by my side.

Danny Korman and Park + Vine for friendship and sustenance, as well as your immeasurable influence on veganism.

The BSM and other cycling/running/yoga buddies, whose appetites inspired this book!

No Meat Athletes everywhere, for putting in the work it takes to do what you do and for letting us be a part of your journey. You inspire me to keep going—thank you!

Note: Page references in
italics indicate photographs.

MATT FRAZIER is an author, entrepreneur, and vegan ultramarathoner, best known as the founder of the No Meat Athlete movement.

Matt's work has been featured in books including Rich Roll's *Finding Ultra*, Brendan Brazier's *Thrive Foods*, Seth Godin's *What to Do When It's Your Turn*, and Heather Crosby's *YumUniverse*; print magazines such as *Runner's World*, *Trail Runner*, and *Canadian Running*; and online publications including the *Huffington Post*, *Forbes*, *Business Insider*, WebMD, *Shape*, and *Competitor*. His first book, *No Meat Athlete: Run on Plants and Discover Your Fittest, Fastest, Happiest Self*, has sold over 25,000 copies, and in 2015 Matt was recognized by Greatist as one of the 100 Most Influential People in Health and Fitness.

Matt works full-time on his business, No Meat Athlete, in Asheville, North Carolina, where he lives with his wife and two children.

STEPFANIE ROMINE is a writer, yoga teacher, and health coach. She's also a no-meat athlete who's into Ashtanga yoga, running half-marathons, and hiking.

With degrees in French and journalism, Stepfanie began her career as a copy editor and reporter. After living abroad and discovering yoga, she turned her passion for healthy living into a career over a decade ago. She now works as a freelance editor and copywriter in the natural products industry, and her bylines have appeared in Greatist, *Eating Well*, *USA Today*, MyFitnessPal, and more. A vegan since 2010 and meat-free since 2006, she shares wellness tips and simple plant-based recipes at theflexiblekitchen.com and around the web.

A yoga teacher since 2009, Stepfanie is certified as a health coach and fitness nutrition specialist through the American Council on Exercise and has studied Ayurveda, herbalism, and holistic nutrition. She is the author of *Cooking with Healing Mushrooms* and has coauthored and written several other wellness titles and cookbooks.

Born and raised in Ohio, she and her husband, Sam, live with their three rescued cats in the mountains outside Asheville, North Carolina.